FAMILY MURDER

Pathologies of Love and Hate

Group for the Advancement of Psychiatry
Committee on Psychiatry and the Law

FAMILY MURDER

Pathologies of
Love and Hate

Edited by

Susan Hatters Friedman, M.D.

Group for the Advancement of Psychiatry
Committee on Psychiatry and the Law

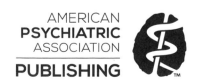

AMERICAN
PSYCHIATRIC
ASSOCIATION
PUBLISHING

If you wish to buy 50 or more copies of the same title, please go to www.appi.org/special discounts for more information.

Copyright © 2019 American Psychiatric Association Publishing

ALL RIGHTS RESERVED

First Edition

Manufactured in the United States of America on acid-free paper

23 22 21 20 19   5 4 3 2 1

American Psychiatric Association Publishing
800 Maine Avenue SW
Suite 900
Washington, DC 20024-2812
www.appi.org

Library of Congress Cataloging-in-Publication Data
Names: Hatters Friedman, Susan, 1975– editor. | American Psychiatric Association Publishing, issuing body.
Title: Family murder : pathologies of love and hate / edited by Susan Hatters Friedman.
Description: First edition. | Washington, DC : American Psychiatric Association Publishing, [2019] | Includes bibliographical references and index.
Identifiers: LCCN 2018026367 (print) | LCCN 2018027030 (ebook) | ISBN 9780873182232 (eb) | ISBN 9780873182225 (pb : alk. paper)
Subjects: | MESH: Homicide—psychology | Family Relations—psychology | Criminals—psychology
Classification: LCC RC569.5.F3 (ebook) | LCC RC569.5.F3 (print) | NLM   WM 605 | DDC 616.85/822—dc23
LC record available at https://lccn.loc.gov/2018026367

British Library Cataloging in Publication Data
A CIP record is available from the British Library.

To our families

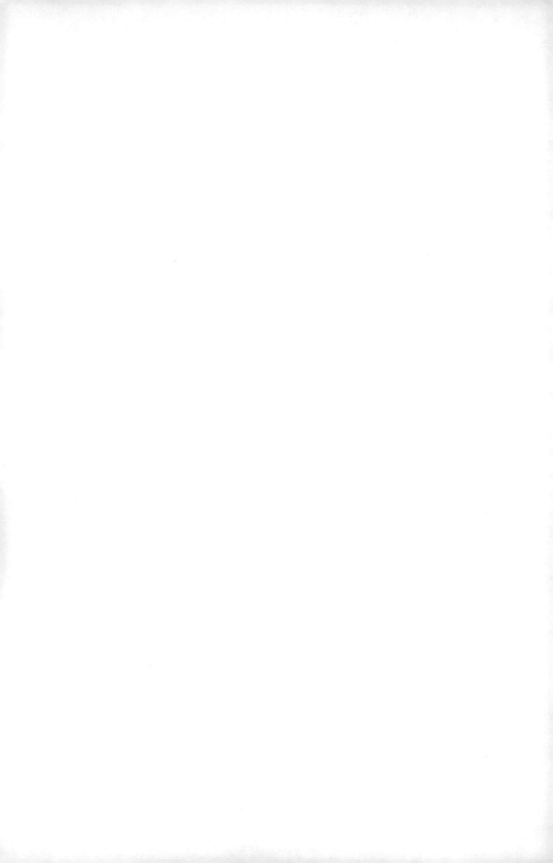

Contents

Contributors

Jacob M. Appel, M.D., J.D., M.P.H.
Assistant Professor of Psychiatry and Medical Education, Mount Sinai School of Medicine, New York, New York

Peter Ash, M.D.
Professor, Department of Psychiatry and Behavioral Sciences, and Director, Psychiatry and Law Service, Emory University, Atlanta, Georgia

Alec Buchanan, M.D., Ph.D., FRCPsych
Professor, Department of Psychiatry, Yale School of Medicine; Associate Chief of Psychiatry, VA Connecticut Healthcare System, New Haven, Connecticut

Susan Hatters Friedman, M.D.
Associate Professor of Psychological Medicine, University of Auckland; Consultant Forensic Psychiatrist, Auckland Regional Forensic Psychiatry Services, Auckland, New Zealand; Professor of Psychiatry, Case Western Reserve University, Cleveland, Ohio

Richard L. Frierson, M.D.
Alexander G. Donald Professor of Clinical Psychiatry and Vice Chair for Education and Director, Forensic Psychiatry Fellowship, Department of Neuropsychiatry and Behavioral Science, University of South Carolina School of Medicine, Columbia, South Carolina

Deborah Giorgi-Guarnieri, J.D., M.D.
President, DGG Medical, Inc.; Private Practice of General and Forensic Psychiatry, Newport News, Virginia

Jacqueline Landess, M.D., J.D.
Assistant Professor of Psychiatry, Department of Psychiatry and Behavioral Neuroscience, St. Louis University, Missouri

Richard Martinez, M.D., M.H.
Robert D. Miller Professor of Forensic Psychiatry and Director, Forensic Psychiatry Training Program, University of Colorado Denver School of Medicine

Debra A. Pinals, M.D.
Clinical Professor of Psychiatry, and Director, Program in Psychiatry, Law, and Ethics, University of Michigan, Ann Arbor

Phillip J. Resnick, M.D.
Professor of Psychiatry, Case Western Reserve University, Cleveland, Ohio

DISCLOSURE OF COMPETING INTERESTS

The following contributor to this book has indicated a financial interest in or other affiliation with a commercial supporter, a manufacturer of a commercial product, a provider of a commercial service, a nongovernmental organization, and/or a governmental agency, as listed below:

Peter Ash, M.D.—*Salary*: Emory University; *Forensic psychiatric consultation*: To attorneys and courts on issues discussed in Chapter 5, "Fatal Maltreatment and Child Abuse Turned to Murder."

The following contributors to this book have indicated no competing interests to disclosure during the year preceding manuscript submission:

Jacob M. Appel, M.D., J.D., M.P.H.
Alec Buchanan, M.D., Ph.D., FRCPsych
Susan Hatters Friedman, M.D.
Richard L. Frierson, M.D.
Deborah Giorgi-Guarnieri, J.D., M.D.
Jacqueline Landess, M.D., J.D.
Debra A. Pinals, M.D.
Phillip J. Resnick, M.D.

Group for the Advancement of Psychiatry Authorship Statement

Each of the chapter authors is a member of the Group for the Advancement of Psychiatry (GAP) Committee on Psychiatry and the Law.

GAP was founded in 1946 under the leadership of Dr. William Menninger. GAP initially was formed after leading military psychiatrists, successful in treating soldiers, returned from World War II and were dismayed with the state of civilian psychiatric care (Deutsch 1959). GAP has been a psychiatric think tank, and members have been keen to advance the field of psychiatry.

GAP's mission statement includes to "offer an objective, critical perspective on current issues facing psychiatry" (Group for the Advancement of Psychiatry 2018). GAP is approximately 300 members strong, and members are organized into various working committees tasked with focusing on issues in psychiatry based on their particular areas of expertise. GAP committee members from across North America meet twice yearly to discuss issues facing the field and to work on GAP projects.

The first GAP report, about electroconvulsive therapy, was published in 1947. The first report by the Committee on Psychiatry and the Law was *Commitment Procedures* (GAP Report No. 4) in 1948, soon followed by *Psychiatrically Deviated Sex Offenders* (GAP Report No. 9) in 1950. In 1954, *Criminal Responsibility and Psychiatric Expert Testimony* (GAP Report No. 26) was published and was later cited in Judge Bazelon's *Durham* opinion (Deutsch 1959).

GAP works are a collective effort of GAP committees. This book represents effort beyond the writing of the individual chapters. Each of the chapter authors has, in addition to writing their chapter, critically reviewed and commented on each of the other chapters. After this process, each chapter is critically reviewed by the members of the GAP Publication Board. So, although each chapter has a listed author, each chapter has also had extensive input from more than a dozen members of GAP.

REFERENCES

Deutsch A: The Story of GAP. New York, Group for the Advancement of Psychiatry, 1959

Group for the Advancement of Psychiatry: Mission statement, 2018. Available at http://www.ourgap.org. Accessed May 20, 2018.

Introduction

In the autumn of 1994, Susan Smith drowned her two young sons by driving her car into a lake with the boys strapped into their car seats inside. She attempted to conceal the crime and set off a nationwide manhunt for an imaginary black carjacker whom she claimed had kidnapped her children. Over the following week, Susan Smith appeared on national television with her estranged husband, tearfully pleading for the return of the sons, while authorities circulated sketches of the "kidnapper."

The break in the case occurred when Smith's story proved inconsistent with the routine workings of a traffic signal. She had claimed that she was stopped at a deserted traffic light when the carjacker, who lay in wait, had commanded her to get out of the car. However, the stoplight at which she claimed to be stopped only turned red if triggered by opposing traffic. Yet no one had witnessed the carjacking.

Smith confessed 9 days later, after the local police chief told her they had a videotape of that street because of drug trafficking surveillance. News stories and commentaries changed from treating her as a struggling young mother beset with tragedy to a most evil killer. America wondered, "How could she?" Smith was eventually sentenced to life in prison and will be eligible for parole in 2024 (Gardner 2015).

We have all heard or read about cases in the media—distinct from our professional roles—that touched us deeply. The poignancy of these cases proved particularly striking for me as I was coming of age. Two such crimes are branded indelibly in my memory: the Susan Smith case and the O.J. Simpson/Nicole Brown Simpson case.

Susan Smith was a young mother, like myself, and she shared my first name. With America's most common surname, Smith, she could be everywoman. Initially, I watched with the rest of the country as we wondered about this "black man" and where and why he would have taken her children. The news also touched on my deepest fears. What young mother does not fear harm befalling her children or her children being taken?

What draws the line between a mother who could kill her children (and even successfully, albeit temporarily, cover up the crime while appearing daily on national television) and "the rest of us"? This was not the usual plot of mystery novels. Reading those books was always about figuring out who the guilty "other" was, rather than the unthinkable—parents killing their own children.

Yet the danger from within the family has been the theme of fairy tales since time began. Snow White's jealous stepmother ordered a huntsman to kill her fairer stepdaughter and bring back her heart as proof. Hansel and Gretel's evil stepmother was the one with the idea of taking the children deep into the forest. There was a famine, and she convinced their father that abandonment was the best plan so that the adults could eat the limited food supply. Stepmothers predominate as villains, but one must keep in mind that stepmothers were more common in centuries past because of high maternal mortality rates. An old French proverb about stepfathers went so far as to say: "*Quand la femme se remarie ayant enfants, elle leur fait un ennemi pour parent*" ("The mother of babes who elects to re-wed has taken the enemy into her bed").

A few months before the Susan Smith case, in June 1994, another alleged family murder had occurred that also became front page news across the United States. Nicole Brown and her friend Ron Goldman had been stabbed to death outside her home (ABC News 2014). They were allegedly murdered by football legend O.J. Simpson, Brown's ex-husband. Goldman had stopped by Brown's residence to drop off sunglasses accidentally left at the restaurant where he worked. Brown and Goldman were viciously killed. A history of a tumultuous jealous marital relationship came out, as well as a fear that Brown reported to friends—that Simpson was stalking her and that he would kill her if he found her with another man.

In 2016, a highly acclaimed FX series entitled *The People v. O.J. Simpson: American Crime Story* reexplored the "trial of the century" (Murphy 2016). Back when the case was in the news daily, it pervaded American culture. If the speculation about the crime were true, people asked, how could a nationally treasured football hero just suddenly murder his ex-wife? And why? How could someone so important be so jealous of his ex that he felt compelled to stalk and kill her? O.J.'s high-powered attorneys used a catchphrase about a bloodied glove with the victims' DNA: "If it doesn't fit, you must acquit." Simpson was eventually acquitted in his controversial criminal trial, yet many doubted his innocence. In civil court, he was ordered to pay $33.5 million for the pair's wrongful death. In a later 2008 case, O. J. Simpson was found guilty of 12 charges, including kidnapping, robbery, and assault with a deadly weapon; he was released on parole in late 2017 (Kreps 2017).

In most violence and homicide, the perpetrator is male. Yet, in family violence, these numbers are different. Violence by women occurs *primarily* within the family. Additionally, family violence is not distinct to our society or even to human beings alone. There is much to learn from family murders both historically and in the animal kingdom. Some of the same primal feelings or needs are the underpinnings. The motives are often simple emotions that everyone experiences—jealousy, greed, pride, anger, desire for revenge—but, hopefully, distinctly out of proportion to our own personal experiences of the same emotions.

Cases of murder within the family make for frequent media headlines. They fascinate the nation. The family is considered the most sacrosanct place of comfort. Why would one family member kill another? Violence and homicide within the family are public health issues. Indeed, violence within the family is a topic that mental health professionals hear of all too often in clinical practice. Yet little information is presented about commonalities between these tragedies. There is a dearth of guidance in the research literature for mental health professionals who treat these families and the child protection workers and lawyers who interact with them. How can we differentiate which cases will become future murder cases and help prevent this? How can we intervene? This book's unique approach in discussing the various types of family murder—the commonalities and differences and society's misconceptions—is designed to serve as a comprehensive guide to these tragedies, from risk factors and prevention to unique treatment issues and the aftermath.

In this book, high-profile media cases serve as starting points to consider each different category of family murder. How like us or unlike us is the alleged perpetrator? More often than seeing differences, we see similarities and recognize a shared humanity. This book brings together the current psychiatric understandings of different forms of murder within the family, utilizing both cases and research data. The epidemiology and public health implications and the various motivations for the subtype of family murder are explicated. Unique assessment issues (e.g., risk assessments, sanity evaluations), as well as the aftermath, sentencing, and working with perpetrators, are described. This critical information, gathered in one place, should help mental health practitioners with management and prevention, as well as those working in the criminal justice arena.

Each chapter focuses on one type of murder in the family. Beginning with partnership, this book progresses through the life cycle of the family. The volume begins by focusing on *homicides within the intimate partner relationship.* Although the Nicole Brown Simpson case discussed earlier may immediately come to mind for many, violence is not unidirectional, and women, too, kill their partners. Some women kill for the same reasons as their male counterparts—explosive jealousy, anger in the context of a violent relationship, and so forth—but other patterns emerge as well—such as the battered woman who in a single act kills her abuser or the "black widow" who kills for money. These types of cases merit their own consideration.

Progressing through the life of a family, then, the text next turns to *feticide*, the (nonabortion) purposeful killing of a fetus during the woman's pregnancy. Two very different scenarios emerge: the mother's paramour kills the unwanted fetus or the (nonmother) female perpetrator who "needs" a baby yet cannot have one of her own accidentally kills the fetus while attempting to rip it from the mother's womb. Also, women may unintentionally miscarry due to substance misuse. The book then moves on to *neonaticide,* the term coined by Dr. Phillip Resnick (1970) to describe murder of the infant in the first day of life. Neonaticide is almost always perpetrated by the mother acting alone after hiding or denying her pregnancy. Society is shocked to learn of cases when abandoned neonates are found in garbage bins or exposed to the elements, yet no one knew of the very existence of the pregnancy. Next, the book turns to the more general filicide: *murder of one's children.* While mothers such as Susan Smith have killed their children in singular lethal events, death as an end result of chronic abuse or neglect by a parent is much more common and is described.

Siblicide, the murder of one's brother or sister, is rare. Yet aggression toward a sibling (hopefully minor during childhood) is epidemiologically the most common type of violence for any of us to have ever perpetrated or experienced. So, what is it that makes some cases go on to murder?

Parricide, the murder of one's parent, is also fortunately rare. Yet the childhood rhymes about Lizzie Borden recounted a real event—she faced trial for the 1892 axe murders of her father and stepmother. *Heavenly Creatures* (Jackson 1994) was similarly based on a true story. In addition, the Menendez brothers' highly publicized 1994 trial for the

Beverly Hills murder of their parents had America wondering about sexual abuse and big money (Ehrlich 2017) and has recently been turned into a miniseries in the *Law & Order* franchise (Balcer 2017).

Next, we turn to consider *intimate partner homicide among the elderly*. Most perpetrators are aging husbands—but the motive is not always the euthanasia-type mercy killing that one hears about from the media. Many are the end result of long-standing intimate partner violence. Finally, *familicide*, in which the entire family is annihilated, is discussed. Every few months there is a case in the national news—these reports may begin with queries of a stranger killing in the context of home invasion. Later, it is reported that it was a killer from within the family, ending with everyone asking why and wondering how warning signs were missed.

We hope that you will find the tragic cases discussed in this volume a compelling jumping off point for further discussions. The authors are forensic psychiatrists who have devoted much of their professional lives to understanding what leads to murder in the family. In the course of our work, we have interviewed hundreds of persons who have killed within the family, as well as thousands of those who have been affected by family violence. While these offenders occasionally fit society's picture of the coldhearted psychopath, more often they are family members dealing with seemingly insurmountable stresses, problems with the family's functioning that significantly predated the murder, and mental illness or substance misuse. We share the data and our insights with the reader in hopes of stimulating further understanding for the victims and for the offenders. Only then can we move toward improved prevention of these family tragedies.

Susan Hatters Friedman, M.D.

REFERENCES

ABC News: O.J. Simpson trial: where are they now? ABC News, June 12, 2014. Available at: http://abcnews.go.com/US/oj-simpson-trial-now/story?id=17377772. Accessed February 1, 2017.

Balcer R (creator): Law & Order True Crime: The Menendez Murders (television series, NBC). Universal City, CA, Universal Television, 2017

Ehrlich B: How the Menendez brothers' trial changed America. Rolling Stone, January 4, 2017. Available at: http://www.rollingstone.com/culture/how-the-menendez-brothers-trial-changed-america-w458897. Accessed February 1, 2017.

Gardner J: "I am not the monster society thinks I am": child killer Susan Smith who murdered her young sons and feigned their kidnap by a black man tries to explain herself on 20th anniversary of her life sentence. Daily Mail, July 22, 2015. Available at: http://www.dailymail.co.uk/news/article-3171009/ I-not-monster-society-thinks-Child-killer-Susan-Smith-murdered-young-sons-feigned-kidnap-black-man-tries-explain-20th-anniversary-life-sentence.html. Accessed February 1, 2017.

Jackson P (dir): Heavenly Creatures (film). Wellington, New Zealand, Wingnut Films, 1994

Kreps D: O.J. Simpson released from prison. Rolling Stone, Oct 1, 2017. Available at: http://www.rollingstone.com/culture/news/oj-simpson-released-from-prison-w506350. Accessed November 22, 2017.

Murphy R (dir): The People v O.J. Simpson: American Crime Story (television series). Los Angeles, CA, FX Network, 2016

Resnick PJ: Murder of the newborn: a psychiatric review of neonaticide. Am J Psychiatry 126(10):58–64, 1970

1

Intimate Partner Homicide by Men

Alec Buchanan, M.D., Ph.D., FRCPsych

INTRODUCTION

Oscar Tejeda, a Cuban man in his mid-40s, shot and killed his girlfriend, Clarinda Garcia, who was in her early 30s. The circumstances are described by Websdale:[1]

> The doctor who was called to the scene noted that Clarinda had bruises around both eyes, three bite marks on her upper torso, a large amount of blood under her head, and blood trickling from her left ear. There were numerous cigarette butts around the room. The motel clerk remembered selling Oscar Tejeda a pack of Marlboros before the killing. The two men conversed in Spanish, and Oscar told him that he would be leaving the motel in 15 or 20 minutes. A maid overheard the conversation between Oscar and Clarinda in the minutes before the killing. Clarinda, speaking in Spanish, was apparently crying. The maid reported that she said, "Papi, I swear to you that it was not me, ask Anton that it was not

[1]Reprinted from Websdale, N: *Understanding Domestic Homicide.* Boston, MA, Northeastern University Press, 1999, pp. 85–87. ©1999 by Neil Websdale. Used with permission.

me. I was not there." Clarinda's sister identified Oscar from photographs police showed her. She told them that he was the man who hit her sister over the head with a gun a couple of weeks earlier....

Clarinda's former boyfriend of five years, Anton Torres, informed officers that he last saw her two days before the murder. He said that the two of them had talked of getting back together.... Oscar said he and Clarinda had been dating for several months.... Two days before the killing, he... invited her to the Miami Motel. There, he noticed a bruise on one of Clarinda's thighs. This upset him and made him extremely jealous. His mood worsened when Clarinda refused to tell him how she suffered the bruise. Oscar went on to say that the two argued and he hit her....

He told investigators he returned to the room without notice, about 30 minutes after leaving, to bring Clarinda breakfast since she had nothing to eat. There he found a Latino man sitting on the bed next to her... again, he beat Clarinda. Oscar remarked to one of the detectives, "You know how women are, they try to brainwash you." After the last beating Clarinda apparently pulled a gun that she kept in her purse and pointed it at Oscar. He told her to "go ahead and shoot me".... On the morning of the murder they... snorted some cocaine. Oscar told detectives that as he was snorting Clarinda warned him, "Keep snorting cocaine and this will soon come to an end."... He continued to carry the image of the other man sitting beside Clarinda on the bed. She drew the gun on him, but he took it away from her this time. Clarinda began to hug and kiss him. As he was kissing her, Oscar shot her in the head.

OVERVIEW

Wolfgang (1956) described intimate partner killing as the most personalized form of homicide. More than for other killings, a knowledge of the duration and intensity of the relationship between victim and offender is crucial to understanding what happened. Society's response has varied over time and according to whether the perpetrator has been male or female. In the Middle Ages, the killing of a wife by her husband was not always treated as a serious offense. At least in England, however, the killing of a husband by his wife was classified as *petit treason,* punishable by burning (Gage 1980).

Although medieval church law had been largely to blame for the discrimination that Gage described, religious movements later contributed to social and legal reforms that provided women with greater protection. The 1641 "Body of Liberties" of the Puritans of the Massachusetts Bay Colony held that, "Everie marryed woeman shall be free from bodilie correction or stripes by her husband, unless it be in his owne defence upon her assault" (Pleck 1987, pp. 21, 22). In the nineteenth century, religious organizations, often supported by the temperance movement, founded the first U.S. refuges for victims of spousal assault.

Many nineteenth-century advances in the treatment of women proved temporary, however (Pleck 1983). Only since the latter half of the twentieth century has violence against intimate partners been consistently regarded both as a criminal act and as a social and public health problem. The "battered women" movement of the 1970s grew largely out of the work of women's groups formed only in the previous decade (Hilton 1989).

In this chapter, I review the literature on male-perpetrated intimate partner homicide and describe assessment issues for clinicians and the role of the criminal justice system. I also review suggestions as to how the frequency of such killings might be reduced.

EPIDEMIOLOGY OF MALE-PERPETRATED INTIMATE PARTNER HOMICIDE

Modern homicides occur more often within marriage than within any other type of family relationship (Wallace 1986). Intimate partner homicide by men is almost always perpetrated against women: of 2,325 intimate partner homicides in Chicago between 1965 and 1993, only 46 occurred in domestic homosexual relationships (Block and Christakos 1995). Women constitute a quarter of all homicide victims in the United States (Fox and Zawitz 2004).

How many of these women are killed by intimate partners is unclear because official classifications do not include ex-partners, who are responsible for approximately 20% of intimate partner homicides (Campbell 1992; Langford et al. 1998). When researchers have gone beyond official statistics to review police files they have found that 40%–50% of women victims are killed by past or present male partners (Campbell 1992; Campbell et al. 2003; Moracco et al. 1998; Wallace 1986). The proportion has changed little since the 1950s (see Wolfgang 1956). If the police data are correct, then intimate partner homicides committed by men account for approximately 1,500 of the 14,000 homicides each year in the United States.

As with all types of violent crime, the burden of these killings falls most heavily on groups that are already disadvantaged. African American, Native American, and Alaskan Native women are disproportionately at risk (Campbell 2007). In 2014, homicide was the second most common cause of death among African American women ages 15–24 years (Centers for Disease Control and Prevension 2014) and the third most common cause of death among Native American women ages 20–24. The racial disparities seem to be explained by differences in socioeconomic status, not ethnicity (Centerwall 1995).

Perpetrators and victims tend to be young (Websdale 1999). The incidence is highest in the early years of relationships and increases with the age difference between the partners (Mercy and Saltzman 1989; Wallace 1986). The crime itself is more violent than other killings by males, more often involving multiple blows, knife wounds, or gunshots (Wolfgang 1956). As for domestic violence generally, male-perpetrated intimate partner homicide takes place in private, late at night, and behind closed doors (Wallace 1986). Wolfgang's Chicago study showed that 85% of the homicides took place in the home and often in the couple's bedroom. The next most common site was the kitchen. Roughly equal proportions involved shooting, stabbing, and beating. Provocation was not common: in less than 10% of cases, the woman was the first to handle a deadly weapon or strike a blow (Wolfgang 1956).

The most common mental health problem that is associated with male-perpetrated intimate partner homicide is substance abuse. More than half of men incarcerated for crimes of intimate partner violence have used drugs or alcohol at the time of their crime (Bureau of Justice Statistics 1998). Alcohol is a more common correlate than drug use (Block and Christakos 1995); over 50% of those who killed intimate partners in two Australian states had used alcohol prior to the killing (Easteal 1993). Other mental disorders have been described as playing an important role in a minority of cases and are described in more detail later. Schizophrenia, depression, and delusional jealousy have been described in the rare instances when men have killed their entire families ("familicide"; see Chapter 10 and Cohen 1995).

MOTIVATION AND ETIOLOGY

Comparisons of the Sexes

Dobash et al. (1992) summarized the differences between homicides carried out by husbands and wives:

Men often kill wives after lengthy periods of prolonged physical violence accompanied by other forms of abuse and coercion; the roles in such cases are seldom if ever reversed. Men perpetrate familicidal massacres, killing spouse and children together; women do not. Men commonly hunt down and kill wives who have left them; women hardly ever behave similarly. Men kill wives as part of planned murder-suicides; analogous acts by women are almost unheard of. Men kill in response to revelations of wifely infidelity; women almost never respond similarly, though their mates are more often adulterous. (p. 81)

Whereas women perpetrators typically fear the man's potential to use violence against them, men do not usually feel that their lives are in immediate danger (Wolfgang 1956).

This list of differences has been widely reported and is based on reliable data. Clinically, however, the value of the comparison seems unclear. To contrast male and female perpetrators assumes that there is one type of behavior and that this behavior has at least two subtypes. The second assumption depends on the first. But is killing one's intimate partner one type of behavior? Any list of differences between men and women says little, on its own, about the causes of those differences. Given the self-defensive aspect of many killings by women, it is not clear why the female perpetrators should be contrasted with the perpetrators of more predatory acts. Clinical tasks, particularly those of risk assessment and intervention, usually require an understanding of causation. The causes of male and female intimate partner killings seem to be different.

Studies of Prior Violence

Men who kill intimate partners have much higher rates of prior criminal behavior, especially violent prior criminal behavior, than do the male perpetrators of other killings (Websdale 1999). The homicide usually follows a series of abusive acts. Among male perpetrators of intimate partner homicide in Chicago, 40% had previous arrests for a violent offense (Block and Christakos 1995). In 87% of the Websdale (1999) series of male-perpetrated intimate partner homicide, the woman had experienced at least one violent assault by her killer prior to the one that led to her death. Overall, between two-thirds and three-quarters of killings of women by their partners are preceded by documented intimate partner violence (Campbell 1981).

Assaults by men on women are relatively common, whereas male-perpetrated intimate partner homicide is not. The factors associated with escalation have been summarized by Walker (2000): 1) a high degree of social isolation, 2) long-standing physical abuse, 3) coercion employed by the man as a major form of communication in resolving interpersonal conflicts, and 4) alcohol or drug use. An escalating pattern in the issuance of protective orders has been noted prior to homicide (Websdale 1999), echoing descriptions of escalations in intimate partner violence itself. The limits to the data mean that escalation may be present simply by definition. De-escalations in violence do not end in killings.

The Perpetrator's Perspective

Chimbos (1978) reported that in more than 70% of cases in which the killing of a spouse was preceded by a fight, the perpetrator said that the fight concerned real or suspected extramarital love affairs. Noting that "Jealousy is common, infidelity is common, but... killing is an extreme rarity," however, Mullen and Taylor (2014, p. 371) concluded that while jealousy may be the prime motivation for many acts of male-perpetrated intimate partner homicide, the question of why this individual, on this occasion, used deadly force is still unanswered.

Anger at supposed infidelity (Brisson 1983), sometimes linked with a sense that they are themselves being victimized, is the most common reason that abusive men give for striking their partners. Wallace (1986) notes the following:

> A significant finding of the research into men and separation is the level of resentment, bitterness and victimization experienced by men. A sense of victimization enables men to feel they have been unjustly treated and this may result in their transferring blame to their wives...violence can be viewed as the ultimate expression of a man's perceived power over his wife; it can equally be viewed as a man's admission that indeed he has no such power. (p. 108)

Perpetrators report being upset by demands—for instance, that the victim be allowed more independence—that they perceive as going beyond the boundaries of acceptable gender roles (Barnard et al. 1982).

Linked to anger is a feeling of betrayal described in many perpetrators and not limited to those who have been in long-standing relationships with their victims. Wallace (1986) concluded that once a woman has communicated her desire to leave a relationship, her risk of being killed increases substantially, irrespective of whether she actually does leave. Nearly 60% of victims are either separated, estranged, or in the process of leaving the perpetrator (Websdale 1999). Wilson and Daly's (1993) analysis of the role of separation and estrangement points to the risk of homicide even when the relationship was not previously violent.

One explanation places male-perpetrated intimate partner homicide among a range of techniques that a patriarchal society uses to control women. Another explanation, without emphasizing mental illness, puts greater emphasis on the psychological plight of the perpetrator. One examination of the role of obsessive jealousy argues that the man sees his victim as part of himself and separation, therefore, as a threat to his very identity (Easteal 1993). Barnard et al. (1982) described "sex role threat," in which men perceive intolerable desertion, rejection, and abandonment as the most important reason for such killings. These authors argued that Western cultural images of what it means to be a male leave little psychological space for sensitivity or dependency in men.

Mental Health

Mental illness appears not to be more common in males who kill their intimate partners than in other men with the same sociodemographic characteristics (Websdale 1999). Descriptions of certain psychiatric conditions, nevertheless, recur in the literature. In more than 90% of the Mowat (1966) cases of morbid jealousy and murder, the victim was an intimate partner. Depression (Buteau et al. 1993; Lester 1992; West 1966), particularly when associated with painful and incapacitating physical illness (Allen 1983) and bipolar illness (Websdale 1999), has also been implicated.

Suicide rates offer some insight into the mental states of some perpetrators. Male perpetrators subsequently killed themselves in 20% of Wolfgang's (1956) series. Thirty-six percent of a series of 217 men in New South Wales who killed their partners either attempted or completed suicide (Wallace 1986). The author of the largest studies of homicide-suicide observed that the odds of suicide following a homicide rise significantly if the victim had been in an intimate relationship with the perpetrator (Stack 1997). The majority of men who kill themselves after killing someone else have killed their intimate partners (Allen 1983).

Suicide pacts represent an important subgroup of murder-suicide and usually involve intimate partners. Traditionally, they were interpreted as acts of kindness, but more recent reviewers note that not infrequently there is a history of abuse (Websdale 1999). Stack (1997) characterizes the relationship between perpetrator and victim in such cases not only as frustrated and chaotic but also as marked by jealousy and ambivalence. He describes a dynamic in some perpetrators, "that one cannot live with the other person but cannot live without them either. A separation or threatened separation arouses anger and depression at the same time. The act of homicide overcomes a sense of helplessness. However, the associated depression and guilt over the loss of one's love object result in suicide" (p. 449).

LEGAL ISSUES

Male sexual jealousy is the most common motive for killing in domestic disputes (Daly et al. 1982). Jealousy is common and a normal emotion. Insanity pleas are in any case unusual and rarely successful when entered (Regoli and Hewitt 1996). When the defendant has killed his intimate partner, these facts taken together seem sufficient to explain why jealousy seldom features in a successful psychiatric defense and why most trials result in conviction.

In the presence of delusions of infidelity, jealousy is usually referred to as "pathological" or "morbid." Delusions that rendered a defendant unaware of what he was doing, unaware of the act's wrongfulness, or unable to conform his behavior to the requirements of the law raise the possibility of an insanity defense. A normal belief that one's partner is unfaithful does not constitute a defense to a charge of murder, however, and the "knowledge of wrongfulness" arm of most versions of the insanity defense will not be satisfied by the mere presence of a delusion of infidelity or a related belief, for instance, that the partner is lying about where he or she has been. Instead, pathological beliefs such as these, especially when they are accompanied by other evidence of psychosis, are more likely to contribute to mitigation. Depending on the jurisdiction, such mitigation may result in conviction on a lesser charge, such as manslaughter instead of murder, on grounds of "diminished responsibility" or "diminished capacity."

Even then, defendants often have difficulty in overcoming a court's skepticism:

> This is even more so if the accused is considered to have grounds for suspecting infidelity. Juries know from everyday experience about the anger of betrayal and though they may condemn it, they often assume the vio-

lence of the cuckolded husband is to be expected, rather than so exceptional that resort to the categories of psychiatry is required to explain it. Thorough preparation is essential to explain to a jury how the paranoiac is to be distinguished from the normal individual grappling with infidelity and how a delusion of infidelity is to be separated from the suspicions and convictions of the commonality. (Mullen 1990, p. 830)

The court's skepticism is likely to be even greater if the morbid jealousy is not part of schizophrenia, delusional disorder, or another recognized psychiatric condition.

In addition, using pathological jealousy as a defense tactic carries its own hazards. A long-standing tendency to become jealous or suspicious or to react aggressively to limited provocation and jealousy's relationship to real and understandable grievances are all open to being interpreted as evidence of dangerous and incorrigible character traits that render the defendant a potential risk to any future sexual partner. Such evidence may then be used to justify a longer sentence (see Mullen 1990). Many morbidly jealous defendants have not sought help, complied poorly with treatment, or not improved, further limiting the degree to which a judge or jury can be relied on to be sympathetic.

WORKING WITH PERPETRATORS

For men in psychiatric treatment with a history of violence toward intimate partners, management starts with a thorough history and mental state evaluation. Mullen and Taylor (2014) provide a list of risk factors to be covered in a psychiatric history: past threats, past violence, access to weapons, escalation of violence or jealousy, violent fantasies, depression (especially in the presence of suicidal preoccupation or behavior), substance use, and cultural beliefs and social background assumptions that condone recourse to violence by a male partner. Research on male-perpetrated intimate partner homicide suggests that depression and substance use, of the commonly occurring psychiatric conditions, warrant particular attention in the presence of a history of domestic violence and, particularly, threats to kill.

Pathological jealousy should be looked for and explored if present. Several authors have pointed to the irrelevance of the truth or falsity of a delusion of infidelity in the diagnosis of pathological jealousy. A statement that one's intimate partner is having an affair may be true by coincidence, irrespective of whether the jealous partner has reason to believe it. Instead, a diagnosis of pathological jealousy should usually derive from the lack of logic in the deductions made in arriving at the belief and to the presence of delusional misinterpretation, particularly of visual information (Mowat 1966). Whereas violence in normal jealousy declines with advancing years, the risk of violence in pathological jealousy seems to continue into old age (Mullen and Taylor 2014).

Psychiatrists are sometimes asked to assess men who are involved in legal cases involving domestic violence. Some of these assessments relate to the appropriateness of bail. Here the risk assessment will usually include distinguishing between impulsive and predatory violence and clarifying the role of other factors, including substance abuse and mental illness. Given the high rates of self-harm in perpetrators of intimate partner homicide, the assessment should also focus on suicide risk. One approach is to ask the perpetrator of domestic violence how he would feel if he killed or seriously injured his victim or if he faced a long prison term.

PREVENTION

Police and Criminal Justice

Websdale (1999) attributes a fall in male-perpetrated intimate partner homicide rates in some areas of the United States to improved police visibility and responsiveness in those areas. Even when there is no history of arrest or conviction, the police are often aware of domestic violence. In one study of domestic assault, the police had been called to the same address for a similar incident in the past 6 months in 80% of cases (Websdale 1999). Websdale (1999) attributes a fall in male-perpetrated intimate partner homicide rates in some black communities in the United States to improved police visibility and responsiveness. Some authors have concluded that protective orders have a deterrent effect on future perpetrators (Keilitz et al. 1998), although such orders are frequently broken without legal consequences. Just under one-third of the women in the Websdale (1999) series were killed with a protective order in place.

Although some have noted that visits from police frequently precede worsening acts of violence (Browne 1987), Websdale (1999) found little evidence that the issuance of a protective order had the same effect. Similar arguments concerning unintended consequences surrounded the introduction of women's shelters in the 1970s and 1980s, which some saw as encouraging retaliation against the women who went to them (Greenland 1990). What should happen to male perpetrators of domestic violence after conviction has been debated. Although court-ordered treatment of domestic violence offenders is now widespread, the evidence for its effectiveness is mixed. One study of 193 male domestic violence offenders found that treatment did not reduce the frequency or severity of subsequent violence (Harrell 1998).

Risk Assessment

Many of the elements of causation reviewed here appear in lists of risk factors for use by those seeking to manage cases of domestic violence. The research literature identifies a range of interconnected precursors: escalation; entrapment of the female victim; separation, estrangement, or divorce of the couple; obsessive possessiveness or morbid jealousy; threats to kill; prior involvement of the police or other agencies; a prior criminal record on the part of the perpetrator; and prior restraining orders (see Websdale 1999).

In this context, *entrapment* refers to the rigid control of a woman's movements, social contacts, money, food, working life, and sexual activities, all resulting from "ongoing coercive control" (Stark and Flitcraft 1995, p. 54). Threats to kill are a long-recognized risk factor (Hart 1988). Male perpetrators of intimate partner homicide are sometimes acting in line with threats made previously concerning what would happen if the woman left (Wilson and Daly 1993). Websdale (1999) found threats to kill in 50% of his series of Florida male-perpetrated intimate partner homicide cases. Threats are made in many abusive relationships, however, without resulting in a killing.

Most abused women do not accurately assess their risk of being killed (Campbell 2007). The most common theory underlying efforts at prevention is that some cases of intimate partner violence follow a trajectory of increasing severity that can only be interrupted by treatment of the abuser or the intervention of the courts. It follows that to reduce male-perpetrated intimate partner homicide using this model, either "trajectory" cases have to be identified in advance or all cases of domestic abuse have to be treated in the same way, with early referrals to treatment and prompt judicial intervention when treatment fails. Both tasks, identification of "trajectory" cases and management of the plurality, require an assessment of risk.

Reviews of risk assessment approaches to the assessment of male-perpetrated intimate partner homicide offer cautions similar to those made with respect to risk assessments in mental health: prediction is difficult when base rates are low (Buchanan 2008). It is unusual for men, even physically abusive men, to kill their partners. Many reviews point to the hazards of unguided clinical assessments of risk and advocate the use of structured instruments, at least as adjuncts to clinical judgment. Crucially, they point out that the rarity of male-perpetrated intimate partner homicide means that the risk factors they identify have been identified by studies of assault, not homicide, and that the risk factors for the two categories may not be the same (see, e.g., Hilton and Harris 2007).

Some risk assessment instruments, such as the Spousal Assault Risk Assessment (SARA; Kropp and Hart 2000), are designed to be completed by correctional, mental health, or other trained staff. The items that compose the scale relate to a potential perpetrator's history (past sexual or other assault, weapon use, and substance use), his attitudes toward violence (including minimization of past episodes), and his mental health (asking about suicidal ideation, mania, psychosis, and personality disorder). Other instruments are intended to be completed by women who have been victims of spousal assault. One contains nine risk factors. Five of the nine relate to a potential perpetrator's past behavior (weapon use, threats with a weapon, threats to kill, causing serious injury, and having forced sex), one relates to circumstances (weapon availability), and three relate to mental state (threats of suicide, substance use, and extreme jealousy) (see Campbell 2007).

The present status of such instruments is similar to that of other structured risk assessment instruments currently in use in criminal justice and mental health. On the one hand, the instruments contain lists of risk factors that have been shown capable of being rated reliably. Many of the risk factors have been empirically validated and demonstrated to be associated with violence. Such a list should be helpful to an assessor. On the other hand, given the low base rate of homicide, anybody attempting to use such an instrument to identify those abusive men who will go on to kill will be faced with two options. Neither seems satisfactory.

The assessor can use the checklist, apply a very low cutoff for what they will call "dangerous," and hence have a high likelihood of detecting future violence (high sensitivity). The consequence of using the instrument in this way is that the low cutoff will generate a large number of false positives. Or the assessor can use the instrument with a high cutoff to minimize this problem (high specificity) with the knowledge that there will be many false negatives. The use of these instruments to assess risk in cases of domestic violence is supported by two facts. First, no one has shown that clinicians operating without a structured instrument measure risk any better. Second, while the accuracy of structured risk assessment instruments in predicting violence in domestic abusers is not better than that of similar instruments used in other settings, it is not worse either (receiver operating characteristic, 0.64: see Campbell 2007).

More important than questions of predictive accuracy, however, is the value of identifying a subset of domestic abusers as "high risk." Any perpetrator of domestic violence should be offered treatment, and their victim should have access to a safe place to live. The courts will often be involved, particularly when violence is serious. If those who are identified as being at high risk represent a separate group of physically abusive men whose violence has different correlates and who are differently motivated, then the most appropriate interventions for them may prove to be different also. This has not yet been demonstrated. Until it is, all forms of risk assessment are likely to remain adjuvants to, rather than central components of, attempts to reduce intimate partner homicide.

MENTAL HEALTH INTERVENTIONS

Rates of depression and substance use are so high, and our ability to identify future cases of male-perpetrated intimate partner homicide so limited, that any effect on rates of depression- and substance-related intimate partner homicide will likely be achieved not by specific treatments for those at risk but by general measures that improve mental health services and access to those services. Providers of mental health services should be trained in the risks associated with a history of domestic violence and have access to services for victims. Involvement of the police and criminal prosecution should not prevent potential perpetrators from being able to obtain treatment, including treatment as a condition of probation or in prison.

Mullen and Taylor (2014) suggest that in pathological jealousy, rates of violence are so high that there must be very good—and clearly documented—reasons not to assume that there is a significant risk and to develop a strategy to address that risk. They note that signs of mounting danger are often ignored or played down by a female partner who cannot accept that their loved one poses a risk to them. Hospitalization of the pathologically jealous male partner is sometimes an option. However, in the absence of insight on the patient's part (to support the case for a voluntary admission) or other signs of serious mental illness (to support the case for an involuntary one), hospitalization is unlikely to be a long-term solution. Attempts to detain them may also be seen by those with pathological jealousy as further evidence of the evil machinations of their partner.

Even when delusions of infidelity are absent and the statutory criteria for involuntary admission to hospital or breaching confidentiality are not met, it can be helpful for a mental health clinician to share his or her concerns about the partner's safety with the patient. When delusions are present, antipsychotic medication may reduce tension and pave the way for psychosocial intervention. Temporary physical separation can have a substantial role in reducing risk but is usually difficult for a treatment team to achieve, often because the at-risk partner is as difficult to persuade of the risk as is the jealous one (Mullen and Taylor 2014).

CONCLUSION

Although intrafamilial homicide is the topic of this book, it is not clear that focusing on cases in which the victim is killed will be the most productive approach to understanding intimate partner violence or to developing interventions through which such violence can be reduced. The epidemiological and case series evidence suggests that the killing of intimate partners by men is not usually a pathology located exclusively in the men concerned or in a mental abnormality from which they suffer. Nor does it seem primarily to represent a failure of criminal justice policy, although there are suggestions that more visible and accessible policing can sometimes prevent violence of this type.

Instead, male-perpetrated intimate partner homicide is best seen as part of a broader thread of pervasive and recurrent social problems relating to male dominance of, and violence against, women. The description of Oscar Tejeda's crime at the beginning of this chapter contains hints of extreme jealousy but also an appeal to two male police officers, "You know how women are." The degree to which these recurrent social problems have been highlighted and confronted has varied over the years. It remains to be seen how effective current efforts to treat perpetrators and protect potential victims will be. The evidence for the benefits of police intervention appears stronger than that for the effectiveness of mental health treatment. From a mental health perspective, two things, nevertheless, seem important.

First, although mental illness is not implicated in the majority of cases, in a few the killing is closely related to psychological symptoms, either of pathological jealousy or of depression, and substance abuse is frequent. It is possible that psychiatric management could have a preventive role in some such cases, especially when combined with sound risk assessment. Second, many perpetrators have troubled personalities and live in challenging environments. Suicide rates are high. While clinical involvement need not preclude the involvement of the criminal justice system, it is likely that both potential perpetrators and many of their victims can benefit from psychologically informed social interventions in cases of domestic abuse and, in some circumstances, from mental health treatment.

REFERENCES

Allen NH: Homicide followed by suicide: Los Angeles, 1970–1979. Suicide Life Threat Behav 13(3):155–165, 1983 6673197

Barnard GW, Vera H, Vera MI, et al: Till death do us part: a study of spouse murder. Bull Am Acad Psychiatry Law 10(4):271–280, 1982 7165803

Block C, Christakos A: Intimate partner homicide in Chicago over 29 years. Crime Delinq 41(4):496–526, 1995

Brisson N: Battering husbands: a survey of abusive men. Victimology 6:338–344, 1983

Browne A: When Battered Women Kill. New York, Free Press, 1987

Buchanan A: Risk of violence by psychiatric patients: beyond the "actuarial versus clinical" assessment debate. Psychiatr Serv 59(2):184–190, 2008 18245161

Bureau of Justice Statistics: Violence by Intimates: Analysis of Data on Crimes by Current or Former Spouses, Boyfriends, and Girlfriends (NCJ-167237). Washington, DC, U.S. Department of Justice, March 1998

Buteau J, Lesage AD, Kiely MC: Homicide followed by suicide: a Quebec case series, 1988–1990. Can J Psychiatry 38(8):552–556, 1993 8242530

Campbell J: Misogyny and homicide of women. ANS Adv Nurs Sci 3(2):67–85, 1981 6778373

Campbell J: If I can't have you, no one can: power and control in homicide of female partners, in Femicide: The Politics of Woman Killing. Edited by Radford J, Russell D. New York, Twayne, 1992, pp 99–113

Campbell J: Prediction of homicide of and by battered women, in Assessing Dangerousness. Edited by Campbell J. New York, Springer, 2007, pp 85–104

Campbell JC, Webster D, Koziol-McLain J, et al: Risk factors for femicide in abusive relationships: results from a multisite case control study. Am J Public Health 93(7):1089–1097, 2003 12835191

Centers for Disease Control and Prevention: Leading Causes of Death in Females, 2014. Available at https://www.cdc.gov/women/lcod/2014/black/index.htm. Accessed May 16, 2018.

Centerwall BS: Race, socioeconomic status, and domestic homicide. JAMA 273(22):1755–1758, 1995 7769768

Chimbos P: Marital Violence: A Study of Interspouse Homicide. San Francisco, CA, R&E Associates, 1978

Cohen DA: Homicidal compulsion and the conditions of freedom: the social and psychological origins of familicide in America's early republic. J Soc Hist 28(4):725–764, 1995

Daly M, Wilson M, Weghorst S: Male sexual jealousy. Ethol Sociobiol 3(1):11–27, 1982

Dobash R, Dobash E, Wilson M, et al: The myth of sexual symmetry in marital violence. Soc Probl 39(1):71–91, 1992

Easteal P: Killing the Beloved: Homicide Between Adult Sexual Intimates. Canberra, Australia, Australian Institute of Criminology, 1993

Fox J, Zawitz M: Homicide Trends in the United States: 2002 Update (NCJ-204885). Washington, DC, U.S. Department of Justice, Bureau of Justice Statistics, November 1, 2004

Gage M: Woman, Church and State (1893). Watertown, MA, Persephone Press, 1980

Greenland C: Family violence: a review of the literature, in Principles and Practice of Forensic Psychiatry. Edited by Bluglass R, Bowden P. Edinburgh, Scotland, Churchill Livingstone, 1990, pp 529–541

Harrell A: The impact of court-ordered treatment for domestic violence offenders, in Legal Interventions in Family Violence: Research Findings and Policy Implications (NCJ-171666). Washington, DC, U.S. Department of Justice, 1998, pp 73–74

Hart B: Beyond the "duty to warn": a therapist's "duty to protect" battered women and children, in Feminist Perspectives on Wife Abuse. Edited by Yllo K, Bograd M. Newbury Park, CA, Sage, 1988, pp 234–248

Hilton Z: One in ten: the struggle and disempowerment of the battered women's movement. Can J Fam Law 7:313–335, 1989

Hilton Z, Harris G: Assessing risk of intimate partner violence, in Assessing Dangerousness. Edited by Campbell J. New York, Springer, 2007, pp 105–125

Keilitz S, Hannaford P, Efkeman H: The effectiveness of civil protection orders, in Legal Interventions in Family Violence: Research Findings and Policy Implications (NCJ-171666). Washington, DC, National Institute of Justice, U.S. Department of Justice, 1998, pp 47–49

Kropp PR, Hart SD: The Spousal Assault Risk Assessment (SARA) guide: reliability and validity in adult male offenders. Law Hum Behav 24(1):101–118, 2000 10693321

Langford L, Isaac N, Kabat S: Homicides related to intimate partner violence in Massachusetts. Homicide Stud 2(4):353–377, 1998

Lester D: Why People Kill Themselves. Springfield, IL, Charles C Thomas, 1992

Mercy JA, Saltzman LE: Fatal violence among spouses in the United States, 1976–85. Am J Public Health 79(5):595–599, 1989 2705594

Moracco K, Runyan C, Butts J: Femicide in North Carolina, 1991–1993: a statewide study of patterns and precursors. Homicide Stud 2(4):422–446, 1998

Mowat R: Morbid Jealousy and Murder. London, Tavistock, 1966

Mullen P: Morbid jealousy and the delusion of infidelity, in Principles and Practice of Forensic Psychiatry. Edited by Bluglass R, Bowden P. Edinburgh, Scotland, Churchill Livingstone, 1990, pp 823–834

Mullen P, Taylor P: Pathologies of passion and related antisocial behaviours, in Forensic Psychiatry: Clinical, Legal and Ethical Issues, 2nd Edition. Edited by Gunn J, Taylor PJ. Boca Raton, FL, CRC Press, 2014

Pleck E: Feminist responses to "Crimes Against Women," 1869–1896. Signs 8(3):451–470, 1983

Pleck E: Domestic Tyranny: The Making of Social Policy Against Family Violence from Colonial Times to the Present. New York, Oxford University Press, 1987

Regoli R, Hewitt J: Exploring Criminal Justice: The Essentials. Sudbury, MA, Jones & Bartlett, 1996

Stack S: Homicide followed by suicide: an analysis of Chicago data. Criminology 35(3):435–453, 1997

Stark E, Flitcraft A: Killing the beast within: woman battering and female suicidality. Int J Health Serv 25(1):43–64, 1995 7729966

Walker L: The Battered Woman Syndrome, 2nd Edition. New York, Springer, 2000

Wallace A: Homicide: The Social Reality. Sydney, Australia, NSW Bureau of Crime Statistics and Research, Attorney General's Department, August 1986

Websdale N: Understanding Domestic Homicide. Boston, MA, Northeastern University Press, 1999

West D: Murder Followed by Suicide. Cambridge, MA, Harvard University Press, 1966

Wilson M, Daly M: Spousal homicide risk and estrangement. Violence Vict 8(1):3–16, 1993 8292563

Wolfgang M: Husband-wife homicides. Journal of Social Theory 2:263–271, 1956

2

Intimate Partner Homicide by Women

Deborah Giorgi-Guarnieri, J.D., M.D.

INTRODUCTION: A MODERN DAY BLACK WIDOW KILLER

In 2007, after 2 years of collecting evidence, investigators procured the arrest of Stacey Castor. Her charges included second-degree murder of her husband, David Castor, and attempted murder of her daughter, Ashley Wallace. During the trial, the media referred to Stacey as "The Black Widow." Just as female black widow spiders devour the males after mating, black widow killers consume their husbands' identities or assets after murdering them. An early article (Munro 2007, p.1) mused,

> If what is said of her is true, Stacey Castor committed the perfect murder when she dispatched her first husband by dosing [sic] him with antifreeze seven years ago.
>
> Her mistake was to repeat it five years later with her second husband, passing it off as suicide.
>
> She then set up her daughter to "confess" to killing both men.

Two years earlier, in August 2005, Stacey Castor called police in Clay, New York, and reported that her husband had locked himself in the bedroom the previous day. She claimed that she had tried to reach him all day while she worked at their business but that there was no answer. She added that he suffered with depression and there was a gun in that room. When police entered the bedroom, they found lifeless, naked David Castor lying on the bed. Next to the bed sat glasses containing apricot brandy, cranberry juice, and antifreeze. Stacey responded with shock when she was told of her husband's death, and she could not be consoled (Chambers 2009).

At the crime scene, investigators found some inconsistencies. Antifreeze can take up to 72 hours to cause death, the three fingerprints on the glass of antifreeze belonged to Stacey, and there was a turkey baster with antifreeze odor in the kitchen trash. Investigators ordered an autopsy that showed "there were crystals[,] and the presence of those crystals in the kidney confirmed that he'd died of ethylene glycol toxicity" (Chambers 2009). The exhumation of the body of Castor's first husband, Michael Wallace, also demonstrated death by antifreeze poisoning. Suspicion rumbled. Fingers pointed toward Stacey Castor. Detectives from the Onondaga County Sheriff's Department questioned her, and she panicked (Battiste 2009).

"The Black Widow" then spun the investigation toward blaming her own daughter, Ashley Wallace. Ashley entered the investigation on her first day of college in September 2007 when investigators visited Ashley and informed her that her stepfather had been murdered. Ashley then called her mother. Stacey invited Ashley for drinks 2 days in a row. On the second day, Ashley's drink tasted "nasty." Seventeen hours after drinking the nasty-tasting alcoholic beverage, Ashley's sister found her comatose in bed. When the paramedics arrived, Stacey handed them a suicide note found next to Ashley's bed. In the suicide note, Ashley confessed to killing her father and stepfather. She barely survived: the physicians surmised that the painkillers from the "nasty" drink would have killed Ashley if she had been found just minutes later. When Ashley woke up, she denied writing the suicide note as well as confessing to killing her father and stepfather. The last thing she remembered was drinking with her mother (Bovsun 2016).

Investigators also looked into the changes in David Castor's will. Stacey changed her husband's will to disinherit his son from his previous marriage and to leave everything to her. Two friends later admitted to falsely witnessing the changes to David Castor's will (Dowty 2014). Those changes in the will helped establish the motive of monetary gain.

On September 14, 2007, Stacey Castor was charged with the murder of David Castor. District attorneys based the accusations on the following facts: the cause of death was antifreeze ingestion, the murder weapons were a turkey baster and a glass, the victim never touched the turkey baster or the glass, friends admitted that they falsely acknowledged David Castor's will, and the motive was inheritance of the estate and insurance monies (Chambers 2009).

At trial, Ashley Wallace testified first. The prosecution presented additional evidence to support their accusations, including wiretaps allowing the jury to hear typing noises that corresponded to the date and time that Ashley allegedly wrote her suicide note on the computer while Stacey was talking on the phone and Ashley was not home as well as inconsistencies in Stacey's statements about Ashley's mental illness. The prosecution further introduced evidence that Stacey also killed her first husband, Michael Wallace (Associated Press 2009).

The defense tried to create reasonable doubt. Stacey Castor, her mother, and Michael Wasielewski (Ashley Wallace's former boyfriend) testified about Ashley's mental instability. Castor alluded to her daughter's depression and suicidal thoughts. Stacey's mother testified that David Castor inappropriately touched Ashley, but the judge instructed the jury to disregard the statement. Wasielewski talked about Ashley's dislike for her stepfather and her contemplation of suicide (O'Hara 2009b). A pharmacology expert explained the blood results estimated Ashley Wallace drank alcohol at midnight and took Ritalin at about 4 A.M., suggesting she was conscious at 4 A.M. The prosecution placed her in bed unconscious at those times (O'Hara 2009a).

The defense did not succeed. In February 2009, Stacey was found guilty of one count of murder in the second degree and one count of attempted murder in the second degree. On March 5, 2009, she was sentenced to up to 54 years in prison and could not request parole for 51 years (Dowty 2016). The court confirmed the media speculations that Stacey Castor was a modern-day black widow killer.

After the verdict, Stacey Castor maintained her innocence in press interviews. She continued to point the finger at her daughter, Ashley. She argued that her trial was unfair and that the judge did not let in the evidence that would exonerate her (Dowty 2013). Her appeals expired in 2015. In the early morning on June 11, 2016, Stacey Castor died in Bedford Hills (Dowty 2016).

OVERVIEW

Throughout history, few women have been known to kill their intimate partners. Society and the law struggle to understand why these women killed. Over time, the media and scholars have placed these women in several categories: abused women isolated from help, women with substance abuse issues, women in the social role of men, elderly women who are overwhelmed caretakers, women with mental health issues, and so-called black widows. Late eighteenth- and early nineteenth-century criminal justice studies of women who kill first noted these patterns and the associated reduced or absent sentences for the homicides: often life situations and mental health were taken into account (Addington and Perumean-Chaney 2014; Callahan 2013). As recently as 2015, media portrayals continue to categorize female killers on a continuum ranging from self-interest to altruism or in the general categories of "the bad," "the mad," or "the sad" (Easteal et al. 2015).

The news media greatly influence society's understanding of the woman who kills her intimate partner. Given the rarity of female killers, the media often sensationalizes the story, focuses on select evidence, and then assigns a speculative motive to the woman. This media tactic, known as *framing*, emphasizes certain aspects and concurrently obscures pertinent factors of the case (Easteal et al. 2015). This allows journalists to use the pathos associated with the domestic environment of the woman to produce social empathy, or lack thereof, in their portrayal of the killer (Reese 2007). In turn, journalists influence the legal system and jurors deliberating a case. Both the media and the law laud some but condemn other women who kill their intimate partners (Easteal et al. 2015).

As contrived and arbitrary as this appears, other countries similarly approach women who kill intimate partners. A study in Canada, noting its differences from previous studies, disclosed that about 25% of women who killed their spouses were previously victims of spousal abuse; less than 50% had mental illness, excluding substance abuse; and very few had prior legal problems (Bourget and Gagné 2012). An Australian study discussed how women who kill their intimate partners experience one or more sources of strain, including victimization, isolation, loss of identity, fear, or desperation (Eriksson and Mazerolle 2013).

The current global understanding of women who kill intimate partners is consistent and has not strayed far from the late eighteenth-century theories.

EPIDEMIOLOGY AND PUBLIC HEALTH PERSPECTIVES

The percentages of females who kill in the United States have always been small and show a significant decrease since 1976. The numbers decreased approximately 40% from 3.1 per 100,000 in 1979 to 1.3 per 100,000 in 1998. Between 1976 and 1997, male victims of intimate partner homicide numbered 18,000 compared with female victims totaling 29,000. Black male victims decreased by 45% and white male victims by 44% during this period (Greenfeld and Snell 2000). The overall percentage of male victims continues to fall: from 10% in 1980 to 5% in 2008 (CNN Library 2016; see also https://www.speakcdn.com/assets/2497/male _ victims_of_intimate_partner_violence.pdf and https://www.bjs.gov/content/pub/pdf/htus8008.pdf).

A 2012 U.S. study reviewed 117 cases of intimate partner murder in Denver, Colorado, between the years 1991 and 2009. Twelve cases, or approximately 10%, were females who killed male partners. The male victims' histories of domestic violence greatly exceeded the female offenders' histories (Belknap et al. 2012). Specifically, Belknap et al. (2012) found "men killed by women were more than seven times as likely to have a prior domestic violence conviction, and more than three times as likely to have a prior domestic violence arrest, compared with women killed by men" (p. 372). These findings again demonstrate the small numbers of female offenders in intimate partner homicides and suggest the most common motive is self-defense.

The American Psychological Association brochure on intimate partner violence includes facts about women who commit murder/suicide or severe violence against their intimate partners. Intimate partners commit approximately 74% of murder/suicides, and only 5% are female. Women with disabilities are 40% more likely to commit severe intimate partner violence than women without disabilities (American Psychological Association 2017). A related statistic is that women are more likely to kill their spouses than their children (Cooper and Smith 2011).

The predominant theory behind females who commit intimate partner homicide is, as noted above, self-defense. In 1992, Margo Wilson and Martin Daly set out to decipher the U.S. statistic that almost as many women killed their husbands as men killed their wives from 1976 to 1985. By comparing female offenders in the United States with female offenders in Canada, Australia, and Great Britain, the study determined that the high U.S. rates were not due to availability of guns, social change, or the proposed general equalization of male and female violent tendencies. They hypothesized that women committed intimate partner killings when coerced, threatened, and empowered to retaliate against the threats and coercion of their intimate partners (Wilson and Daly 1992). Even when the rates of women who killed their husbands were at their highest, the most common theory was self-defense.

Women who kill their female intimate partners are a small subcategory of female intimate partner homicides. Women kill female intimate partners even less often than women kill male intimate partners. A 2008 study in the United States looked specifically at lesbians who killed their intimate partners. The apparent rarity may be in part due to the secrecy and lack of report of the relationship or the lack of specifics about the relationship during the investigation. In this study, Mize and Shackelford (2008) found lesbian victims accounted for 0.3%, or about 133 of about 54,000 cases, of intimate partner homicide victims over a 25-year period. Similarly, in Gannoni and Cussen's (2014) Australian study, same-sex partners accounted for only 2% of intimate partner murders from 1989–1990 to 2009–2010. Female offenders accounted for 13% of the 2% (or about 0.3%). The leading cause of death was stab wounds (Gannoni and Cussen 2014). U.S. statistics are comparable to global statistics on women who kill female intimate partners.

Global studies have demonstrated trends of decreasing female intimate partner violence that are comparable to those in the United States. In 2013, Stöckl et al. reviewed data from 66 countries pertaining to the global incidence of intimate partner murders. Intimate partners committed 13.5% of all homicides. Female offenders killing male partners constituted about 6.3% of all homicides. Males outnumbered females committing intimate partner homicides in all countries except Panama and Brazil, where the numbers were about equal. The highest incidences of female offenders occurred in high-income countries. These global findings support the need for public policy reform in high-income countries such as the United States.

The public policy issues center around education, prevention, and services. The initial issue is whether or not intimate partner homicides are gender biased, suggesting men primarily murder female intimate partners. If this violence is gender biased, then males are the abusers, and females who kill their intimate partners are the victims that strike back.

If violence is not gender biased, then male and females are equal in executing family violence.

Finally, studies have attempted to develop typologies, albeit unsuccessfully (Stöckl et al. 2013). One 2014 study reviewed data from the 2008 National Incident-Based Reporting System and found male victims of intimate partner killings were more likely to be older, more likely to have an older killer, and more likely to be killed by a weapon, and there was a greater likelihood that alcohol or substance use was involved (Addington and Perumean-Chaney 2014). Again, this might only reflect the female victim's reaction to male violence, making it difficult to identify and distinguish typologies.

MOTIVATIONS AND MENTAL HEALTH

Self-Defense Killings

Self-defense or similarly named motivations arose in the earliest theories about women who kill intimate partners ("the sad"). Self-defense as a motivation is perhaps the most common and most studied motivation. The media portray these women as abused, helpless, irrational, and "insane" from battered woman syndrome (BWS) at the time of the murder (Easteal et al. 2015).

The sad retaliate against abusive male partners. They experience different emotions than do men who kill their female partners. Women kill in self-defense when they experience fear, isolation, desperation, failure, and anxiety (Walker 1989).

Since self-defense is the predominant theory behind female intimate partner homicide, the courts allow testimony about BWS as a legal defense. Psychiatric theories supporting BWS include the strain theory, the concept of learned helplessness, the cycle of violence theory, and post-traumatic stress disorder.

In the *general strain theory*, the characteristics of strain that cause women to kill include magnitude, unjust nature, incentives to commit crimes, and low social control (Agnew et al. 2002). These women suffer extreme emotional, physical, and sexual abuse. Additive strain exists when the male victim threatens child abuse or future lethal actions. The sad feel that they have failed their marriage and children, they have lost their identity, and they are isolated from friends and family. Violence is the only means to survival (Eriksson and Mazerolle 2013).

In the 1970s, BWS became a practical concept in the courtroom. The term *learned helplessness* was used to explain how a victim's repeated attempts and failures to protect herself against the violence led to her perception that she was in unavoidable, grave danger (Walker 1977–1978). In 1984, the *cycle of violence theory* explained how the batterer draws the women back after the violence with attention and apologies (Walker 1984). Recently, BWS has been equated with *posttraumatic stress disorder*. The exposures to the traumas create symptoms such as intrusive thoughts and flashbacks that cause a disproportionate fear and/or response (Walker 1992). However, caution must be exercised because all women do not respond in the same way to their batterer.

The Black Widow

The black widow kills one or more partners with malicious intent. These women represent a specific type of the "bad." The media portray them as man-hating aberrations of womanhood (Easteal et al. 2015). Although rare, black widows permeate every culture and every time period. The stereotypical black widow, if there is one, kills her spouse or partner for monetary gain. Other reasons are revenge or for the comforts and attentions paid to a grieving widow. The home is the usual setting, and typical weapons of choice include poison, suffocation, or drowning. Stabbing and shooting are less common. These women enjoy the attention and sympathy of losing their loved one. Rarely suspected, the black widow kills more than once before getting caught in their own web (Anthes 2015).

"The bad" also include female serial killers and women with intent to kill. The media similarly sensationalize female serial killers. "Lady killers," include Nannie Doss, Amy Archer-Gilligan, Dorothea Puente, and Bonnie Parker. Female serial killers typically are 20–30 years old, married, Christian, of average intelligence, and middle-class (Anthes 2015). The rare women killers with the traditional intent to kill are all the remaining women who kill, excluding the sad, the mad, "lady killers," and black widows.

Same-Sex Intimate Partner Killings

Same-sex intimate partner murders involve two women currently or previously involved in a homosexual relationship in which one woman kills her intimate partner. Although few in number, these women are found among the bad, the sad, and the mad. Motives in same-sex intimate partner murders are similar to those in heterosexual intimate partner murders. Motives and other reasons include, in order of prevalence, domestic arguments, revenge, jealousy, desertion/termination of the relationship, money, other arguments, mercy killing, and delusions (Gannoni and Cussen 2014). The ratio of very brutal to less brutal killings among lesbian homicides was 50:50, which is higher than the ratio for heterosexual homicides (35:65).

Mentally Ill Killers

On October 10, 2014, stay-at-home mother Rose Marie Uribes shot and killed her husband. She believed that his soul had been taken. She called a relative and then 911. When police showed up at her townhouse, she confessed. Four weeks before the shooting, Uribes's mental health worsened. She heard taunting voices, saw a legless girl floating in her home, thought her family had abandoned her, and felt she was traveling through time. She had been to the local mental health hospital and seen mental health therapists multiple times prior to the shooting. In April 2016, a Newport News, Virginia, judge found Uribes to be not guilty by reason of insanity for the killing of her husband. It was one of only five successful insanity defenses in Newport News in 10 years (Canty 2016).

Psychotic disorders are the most common mental health diagnoses in the infrequently successful insanity defenses. In contrast, psychotic symptoms are rarely characteristic of the mental state of women who kill their intimate partners. When a seemingly benign woman kills her partner, however, the media and the law investigate many mental health diagnoses or explanations. The truly mentally ill women are "the mad."

The mad overlap with the sad and the bad. The media publish many articles about women who kill and almost always raise the question, "Did she suffer from mental illness?" (Anthes 2015). The courts continue to question whether mental illness was a prominent factor in the pretrial proceedings, the trial, and sentencing of all women who kill. Yet sometimes mental health professionals, the media, or the courts called on for clarity struggle to find any diagnosis. In fact, there are no studies that focus solely on mental health diagnoses as an explanation of motive in women who kill partners/ex-partners.

Given the presumption that women who kill have mental disorders, studies have focused on inpatients and inmates with a history of mental illness as well as symptoms of mental illness at the time of the intimate partner homicide. The existing studies focus on the specific issue of intimate partner killing from the forensic data on all women who kill or the rare study that focuses on male and female intimate partner homicide. Comparisons of the data show neither a specific trend in diagnosis as a motive nor repeatable results.

In 1995, Ogle et al. proposed a single empirical theory to explain all female-perpetrated homicides. The theory submitted eight propositions that focused on stress, how women cope with stress, social status, personality, and the triggers that make women strike out in their environments. This theory is meant to address female homicide in a variety of settings that consider structural, social, and cultural circumstances at the time and place of the murder. The authors emphasized the presence of stress but concluded that mental illness did not seem to be an important factor. The dismissal of mental illness as a causative factor or motive in females who kill is contradicted by the populations in inpatient forensic psychiatric facilities and women's mental health wards in prisons.

In contrast to Ogle et al.'s theory, later studies showed that high percentages of female offenders had severe mental disorders. A 2005 U.S. study found 7 females and 21 males who had undergone inpatient forensic psychiatric evaluation after killing their spouses. The results indicated that about half of the study subjects suffered from a psychotic disorder (Farooque et al. 2005). In 2008, a Swedish study reviewed 24 cases of female defendants and compared them with 24 cases of male defendants who had killed their partners/ex-partners (Yourstone et al. 2008). The histories of the defendants showed that

> [m]ore than half of the offenders had notes about some kind of psychiatric problem and/or mental illness. Among these, more than half had previously been in institutional care and/or were in institutional care at the time of the current crime. The remaining part had been or were in noninstitutional care. Many of the offenders had also notes about alcohol, drugs and/or medication abuse. There were no gender differences on any of these variables.... (p. 380)

In this study, 92% of the offenders underwent a forensic psychiatric evaluation or a minor forensic psychiatric assessment. This study did not specify the mental health histories or the specific diagnosis of mental illness at the time of the homicide in the female offenders who had killed their partners.

The studies subsequent to 2010 swung the pendulum back toward Ogle et al.'s deemphasis on mental illness as a causative factor. Flynn et al.'s (2011) study from England and Wales reported that 18% of women had acute mental illness at the time they killed. The cases originated from a mental health data bank. Ten percent of the female offenders had committed intimate partner homicide. The types of mental illness included psychotic, mood, substance use, and personality disorders.

In 2015, Hellen et al. reviewed 10 cases of female homicide offenders (two of the women had killed their husbands) and found mental illness was uncommon in the offenders. The results confirmed that the setting was in the home mostly and that the offenders had no prior convictions and were isolated socially, dependent on the victim, and of low socioeconomic status. Similarly, in 2016, a Swedish study identified nine female offenders of intimate partner homicide (Caman et al. 2016). The authors reviewed five national registries and police reports to identify the women. The women were more likely to be unemployed, to be engaged in substance abuse, and to have been victimized by the victim. Six female offenders were intoxicated at the time of the homicide. Six of the female offenders had at least one previous inpatient psychiatric hospitalization. Their diagnoses were primarily substance abuse and personality disorder. None of the six carried a psychotic disorder diagnosis.

One 2012 study stands out in contrast to the trend since 2010 toward research finding mental illness to be a less important factor in female intimate partner homicide. In a coroner's study, Bourget and Gagné (2012) reported a high prevalence of psychiatric diagnoses in offenders of intimate partner homicides, including personality disorder and psychosis. Forty-two female offenders were included in this Quebec study. The presence of a mental disorder was determined in 19 female offenders: 1 had no mental disorder, 6 had major depressive disorder, 9 were acutely intoxicated, 1 had schizophrenia, and 2 had an unspecified mental disorder. Psychiatric motives presented in 16 (or 42%) of the killings. Psychotic intent was determined in 2 (10%) cases. The study concluded that there were high rates of depression (36%) and intoxication (48%) among female offenders. Although the study numbers were low and the data came from coroners' reports, Bourget and Gagné provided conclusions about mental disorders.

Obviously, the studies complicate the attempts to determine the role that mental illness plays as a motive in the small number of women who kill their spouses/ex-spouses. Perhaps the explanation of the woman's social situation overshadows the role of mental illness in discussing intimate partner killings. Perhaps the role of mental illness should contribute to the social situation in explaining intimate partner killings. With either explanation, more studies focused on mental illness in females who commit intimate partner homicide are needed to understand mental health issues in these domestic cases.

UNIQUE ASSESSMENT ISSUES

The mental state of women who kill partners, whether these women be mad, bad, or sad, is almost always considered in the legal procedure and disposition of the case. Who can forget the mental image of Lorena Bobbitt emerging from her apartment with half of her husband's penis in her hand on her way to tossing it into some random field? She didn't plan it: she just saw the knife on the counter when she went to get a drink of water. John Bobbitt, her husband, was in a deep, inebriated sleep after returning home and raping Lorena, as he had done many times before. After disposing of the severed penis in a field and returning to their apartment, Lorena called 911 and told them what she had done. The Virginia jury in Lorena Bobbitt's case considered the abusive relationship issues and ultimately accepted the diagnosis of depression, finding her not guilty by reason of insanity (Margolick 1994). Some experts consider this case an aberration. The court's ruling, however, was in line with Virginia's unique insanity defense.

The court's ruling was also in line with BWS. The law provides a special self-defense—namely, BWS—or at least allows testimony about the abusive relationship for many of the female defendants who kill their spouses. Female killings account for only 2.8% of male homicide victims (Catalano 2013). Every state in the United States recognizes BWS expert testimony (Kinports 2004). The testimony serves multiple purposes, but the main argument is that BWS creates a state of mind that explains why the crime is one of self-defense (Walker 1992). BWS is considered a form of self-defense that was not accounted for in the traditional American legal system meant for white male defendants. Its inclusion in legal proceedings does not codify BWS as a mental illness, but it does define it as a reasonable use of force in self-defense. Yet many women are denied the defense because juries decide that the defendant did not meet the expert's strict criteria of a battered woman, and some studies suggest that these women receive harsher sentences (Jacobsen and Bex Lempert 2013). As Stallion (2016) asserted,

> Expert testimony regarding BWS should focus on the battered woman who is facing trial, detailing *her* reactions to the abuse she has suffered. To group the traits of all battered women into one single definition is to deprive other women, who similarly faced horrendous abuse, of the ability to claim self-defense. BWS should not be a one-size-fits-all explanation, and it is imperative that an expert present evidence as to why a particular battered woman acted in the particular way that she did. (p. 306)

Stallion coached mental health professionals to understand that BWS is a unique challenge to expert testimony, urging a tailored content in the testimony. Providing expert testimony about a syndrome, not a mental illness, differs from the typical role of a clinician in court.

The courts provide better guidelines for testimony for an insanity defense. Courts prove receptive to using the insanity defense in cases of female intimate partner homicide. In a study of 28 intimate partner killings in Tennessee (21 male and 7 female offenders), the forensic evaluations supported three insanity defenses (11% of the cases): in these three cases, the defendants received diagnoses of psychotic disorders. The courts found nine defendants (32%) incompetent to stand trial (Farooque et al. 2005).

Similarly, Flynn et al. (2011) offered the possibility that offenders of intimate partner homicide could raise the insanity defense. Analysis demonstrated that factors predicting a hospital disposition included the diagnosis of schizophrenia, mental health outcome in court, mental health issues at the time of the offense, recent contact with the mental health system, a victim over the age of 75, and minority race or ethnicity. Sex was not a factor. Flynn et al.'s results documented that 111 of the 160 women who killed a spouse went to prison, 10 went to the hospital, and 39 were released with noncustodial care (Flynn et al. 2011). These numbers suggest that even with expert testimony about mental health conditions, most women went to prison. The study fully supports psychiatric reports for female killers and suggests risk factors that might help develop a risk assessment.

Experts might borrow from their role in insanity defense cases to perform their roles in BWS cases. If the mental state at the time a woman kills her intimate partner is one of self-defense, then the expert can testify about the connection from diagnoses, circumstances, and history of abuse to the act of homicide. This approach would blend the mental health diagnosis with the circumstances of the killing in considering a self-defense motive, allowing the court to see a fuller picture of the mental state of the woman at the time she killed her intimate partner.

AFTERMATH

Whether incarcerated, institutionalized, or in noncustodial care, female defendants cost and pay a huge price. In 2003, the Centers for Disease Control and Prevention estimated that the cost to society from intimate partner violence victimization of women approached $6 billion annually (National Center for Injury Prevention and Control 2003). Estimated costs included those related to shelters, legal system procedures, social services, and medical care.

The Castor case is an example of costly follow-up investigations and legal proceedings. Subsequent to the trial in 2009, the prosecution began investigations into the 2002 death of Stacey's father (Kenyon 2010). In 2010, David Wallace Jr. and his mother brought suit to recover lost money as a result of the fraudulent will (Dowty 2014). Stacey appealed her conviction in 2013 (Dowty 2015). The costs of these investigations, hearings, and appeals accumulated after Stacey's conviction. A 2010 study estimated that the average murder trial costs $17.25 million (DeLisi et al. 2010).

The Bobbitt and Uribes cases are examples of subsequent costs to the state legal and mental health systems. Lorena Bobbitt spent 45 days in a maximum-security hospital and was released. Uribes also underwent a 45-day evaluation in a maximum-security hospital and remains in a minimum-security state mental hospital for treatment until she is deemed to be no longer a risk to society. The daily cost of forensic psychiatric hospitalization in Virginia in 2012 averaged $300 per day. The U.S. average in 2012 was approximately $600 per day (Lutterman 2014). The courts also incur expenses during the hospital assessments and treatments as a result of legally mandated hearings.

Costs that cannot be estimated as a consequence of intimate partner homicides include corollary victims, dissolution of the family, and emotional damage. In 2014, Smith et al. reviewed 4,470 deaths and 3,350 incidents of intimate partner murder. Corollary victims (other family members, friends, acquaintances, or police officers on the scene) accounted for 20% of the deaths. These deaths increase the costs to society. The same systems that interact with the offenders and victims of intimate partner violence could aid in the risk assessment for intimate partner or corollary victim murders (Smith et al. 2014). Prevention would decrease costs.

PREVENTION

The overall number of women who kill intimate partners has been decreasing since the 1970s. Prevention remains an issue because often intimate partner violence precedes intimate partner murders. Female intimate partner homicides occur in very different social and economic environments than do typical killings. Whether the killer is "mad," "bad," or "sad," the killer's social safety net failed (Hellen et al. 2015).

Many of the female offenders' decisions hinge on the immediate emotion and/or setting. Significant numbers of the female offenders come from a background of lower socioeconomic status, domestic violence, and limited support systems. Caman et al. (2016) specifically noted that economic disadvantage usually equated to unemployment, and limited support system promoted dependence on the partner, even if the partner was abusive. The study also emphasized that more than half the female offenders had a history of substance use, and the majority were intoxicated at the time of the killing (Caman et al. 2016). Past emotional experiences combined with current mental state might be the main factor that distinguishes the women who strike back from the women who retreat.

Prevention strategies include intervention in intimate partner violence, laws to remove firearms from homes with intimate partner violence, prevention of intimate partner violence, treatment of mental health issues, and risk assessments (Smith et al. 2014). Risk assessment tools could be developed. A simple checklist could both identify the current level of danger and collect data that could be used to create more accurate risk assessments (van Wormer 2009). The Danger Assessment (Campbell et al. 2009) predicts lethality in intimate partner femicide. van Wormer and Roberts (2008) created the Seven-Stage Crisis Intervention Model to assess a battered woman's risk of losing her life. Similar risk assessment tools could be developed to assess potential female offenders.

Previous studies have indicated that use of a firearm during intimate partner violence results in 12 times the number of deaths in homes with firearms (Saltzman et al. 1992). Some states have implemented laws to allow the removal of weapons from the home of known intimate partner violence (Smith et al. 2014), but the effectiveness of these laws in preventing homicides is unstudied.

Previous intimate partner violence is the strongest predictor of intimate partner homicide (Campbell et al. 2009). Primary prevention programs exist. School programs intend to prevent date violence, and other programs target adult couples (Smith et al. 2014). Alcohol abuse treatments and screenings of individuals in substance abuse treatment programs also are key to prevention (van Wormer 2009). Farooque et al. (2005) noted that a history of partner abuse combined with jealousy or substance abuse predicts fatality. Intervention during intimate partner violence may preempt intimate partner murder.

Police might play an important role in identifying female victims of abuse before females commit intimate partner homicide because females report nonlethal abuse more than males. Intervention, education, and treatment programs for these abused women also might prevent future male intimate partner homicide.

In Estonia, the Ministry of Justice (2015, p. 301) published prevention strategies for 2015–2020:

- Change people's values and attitudes and to influence people not to use violence.
- Reduce the possibility of emergence of such situations that promote violence.
- Improve the access of victims of violence to assisting and support services.
- Ensure the more effective intervention of the criminal justice system to crimes of violence.

These goals reflect interventions that have worked in the past (van Wormer 2009). With better risk assessment tools, resources can be streamlined to prevent intimate partner violence from becoming intimate partner homicide. The already diminishing numbers of female-perpetrated intimate partner deaths may eventually be reduced to zero.

CONCLUSION

Female offenders in intimate partner killings are few and growing fewer. Due to the small numbers, researchers may never accurately capture when and why a woman might fatally strike her intimate partner. Many female offenders have suffered abuse at the hands of their partner. A few female offenders calculate the demise of their partners for monetary gain. Although few women who kill experience mental illness at the time of the offense, many of all types of female offenders have histories of mental illness and deprivation. Despite the small numbers and varied motives, interventions in intimate partner violence have succeeded in decreasing the numbers of women who kill intimate partners. Perhaps, women who kill their intimate partners should be studied for their decreasing rates of killing as well as their reasons for the violence.

REFERENCES

Addington LA, Perumean-Chaney SE: Fatal and non-fatal intimate partner violence: what separates the men from the women for victimizations reported to police? Homicide Stud 18(2):196–220, 2014

Agnew R, Brezina T, Wright JP, et al: Strain, personality traits, and delinquency: extending general strain theory. Criminology 40(1):43–72, 2002

American Psychological Association: Intimate Partner Violence: Facts and Resources. Washington, DC, American Psychological Association, 2017. Available at: http://www.apa.org/topics/violence/partner.aspx. Accessed September 29, 2017.

Anthes E: Lady killers. The New Yorker, May 9, 2015. Available at: https://www.newyorker.com/tech/elements/female-serial-killers. Accessed September 29, 2017.

Associated Press: Woman convicted of poisoning husband, harming daughter. Fox News, February 5, 2009. Available at: http://www.foxnews.com/story/2009/02/05/woman-convicted-poisoning-husband-harming-daughter.html. Accessed September 29, 2017.

Battiste N: (2009, April 22) Exclusive: Mother and Daughter Face Off in Murder Mystery. ABC News. Available at: http://abcnews.go.com/2020/story?id=7389055&page=1. Accessed September 29, 2017.

Belknap J, Larson D, Abrams ML, et al: Types of intimate partner homicides committed by women: self-defense, proxy/retaliation, and sexual proprietariness. Homicide Stud 16(4):359–379, 2012

Bourget D, Gagné P: Women who kill their mates. Behav Sci Law 30(5):598–614, 2012 23015414

Bovsun M: Stacey Castor killed two husbands, tried to murder own daughter and frame her for the deaths. New York Daily News, March 19, 2016

Callahan K: Women who kill: an analysis of cases in late eighteenth- and early nineteenth-century London. J Soc Hist 46(4):1013–1038, 2013

Caman S, Howner K, Kristiansson M, et al: Differentiating male and female intimate partner homicide killers: a study of social, criminological, and clinical factors. Int J Forensic Ment Health 15(1):26–34, 2016

Campbell JC, Webster DW, Glass N: The danger assessment: validation of a lethality risk assessment instrument for intimate partner femicide. J Interpers Violence 24(4):653–674, 2009 18667689

Canty M: Rarely used defense gets wife acquitted in Newport News slaying. Daily Press, September 27, 2016. Available at: http://www.dailypress.com/news/crime/dp-nws-evg-uribes-insanity-defense-20160914-story.html. Accessed September 29, 2017.

Catalano S: Special Report: Intimate Partner Violence: Attributes of Victimization, 1993–2011 (NCJ 243300). Washington, DC, U.S. Department of Justice, Office of Justice Programs, Bureau of Justice Statistics, 2013. Available at: http://www.bjs.gov/content/pub/pdf/ipvav9311.pdf. Accessed September 29, 2017.

Chambers A: "Black widow" Stacey Castor accused in anti-freeze murder. ABC News, April 21, 2009. Available at: https://abcnews.go.com/2020/story?id=7380832&page=1. Accessed September 29, 2017.

CNN Library: Domestic (intimate partner) violence fast facts. CNN, May 4, 2016. Available at: http://www.cnn.com/2013/12/06/us/domestic-intimate-partner-violence-fast-facts/index.html. Accessed September 29, 2017.

Cooper A, Smith E: Homicide Trends in the United States, 1980–2008: Annual Rates for 2009, 2010 (Patterns and Trends, NCJ 236018). Washington, DC, U.S. Department of Justice, Office of Justice Programs, Bureau of Justice Statistics, 2011

DeLisi M, Kosloski A, Sween M, et al: Murder by numbers: monetary costs imposed by a sample of homicide offenders. Journal of Forensic Psychiatry & Psychology 21(4):501–513, 2010

Dowty D: Judge rejects Stacey Castor's claim in appeal that dead husband's estate lawyer represented her in murder probe. Syracuse.com, December 5, 2013. Available at: http://www.syracuse.com/news/index.ssf/2013/12/judge_rejects_stacey_castors_claim_that_dead_husbands_estate_lawyer_represented.html. Accessed September 29, 2017.

Dowty D: Appeals court overturns $377K verdict for victim's son in notorious Stacey Castor murder. Syracuse.com, May 13, 2014. Available at: http://www.syracuse.com/news/index.ssf/2014/05/appeals_court_overturns_375k_verdict_for_victims_son_in_notorious_stacey_castor.html. Accessed September 29, 2017.

Dowty D: Appeals court puts nail in coffin for notorious murderer Stacey Castor's appeal. Syracuse.com, June 8, 2015. Available at: http://www.syracuse.com/crime/index.ssf/2015/06/appeals_court_puts_nail_in_coffin_for_notorious_murderer_stacey_castors_appeal.html. Accessed September 29, 2017.

Dowty D: DA: antifreeze murderer Stacey Castor, who poisoned husband, dead at 48. Syracuse.com, June 11, 2016. Available at: http://www.syracuse.com/crime/index.ssf/2016/06/da_notorious_antifreeze_murderer_stacey_castor_who_poisoned_husband_dead_at_48.html. Accessed September 29, 2017.

Easteal P, Bartels L, Nelson N, et al: How are women who kill portrayed in newspaper media? Connections with social values and the legal system. Womens Stud Int Forum 51:31–41, 2015

Eriksson L, Mazerolle P: A general strain theory of intimate partner homicide. Aggress Violent Behav 18(5):462–470, 2013

Farooque RS, Stout RG, Ernst FA: Heterosexual intimate partner homicide: review of ten years of clinical experience. J Forensic Sci 50:648–651, 2005

Flynn S, Abel KM, While D, et al: Mental illness, gender and homicide: a population-based descriptive study. Psychiatry Res 185(3):368–375, 2011 20724002

Gannoni A, Cussen T: Same-sex intimate partner homicide in Australia. Trends & Issues in Crime and Criminal Justice 469:1–7, 2014

Greenfeld LA, Snell TL: Women offenders. Bureau of Justice Statistics Special Report (Revised Edition), October 3, 2000. Available at: https://www.bjs.gov/content/pub/pdf/wo.pdf. Accessed September 29, 2017.

Hellen F, Lange-Asschenfeldt C, Ritz-Timme S, et al: How could she? Psychosocial analysis of ten homicide cases committed by women. J Forensic Leg Med 36:25–31, 2015 26355562

Jacobsen C, Bex Lempert L: Institutional disparities: considerations of gender in the commutation process for incarcerated women. Signs 39(1):265–289, 2013

Kenyon J: Did Stacey Castor murder her own father? CNYCentral.com, February 1, 2010. Available at: http://cnycentral.com/news/local/did-stacey-castor-murder-her-own-father. Accessed September 29, 2017.

Kinports K: So much activity, so little change: a reply to the critics of battered women's self-defense. St. Louis University Public Law Review 23:155–191, 2004

Lutterman T: Virginia's State Mental Health System: National Comparisons and Trends in State Mental Health Systems. Alexandria, VA, National Association of State Mental Health Program Directors Research Institute, September 9, 2014. Available at: http:// dls.virginia.gov/GROUPS/MHS/va%20system.pdf. Accessed September 29, 2017.

Margolick D: Lorena Bobbitt acquitted in mutilation of husband. The New York Times, January 22, 1994. Available at https://www.nytimes.com/1994/01/22/us/lorena-bobbitt-acquitted-in-mutilation-of-husband.html. Accessed September 29, 2017.

Ministry of Justice: Policing intimate partner violence and the typology of perpetrators. 2015, p 301. Available at: https://repository.mruni.eu/bitstream/handle/007/14994/Traat.pdf?sequence=1. Accessed May 5, 2018.

Mize KD, Shackelford TK: Intimate partner homicide methods in heterosexual, gay, and lesbian relationships. Violence Vict 23(1):98–114, 2008 18396584

Munro I: Black widow. Dominion Post, Oct 13, 2007, p 1

National Center for Injury Prevention and Control: Costs of Intimate Partner Violence Against Women in the United States. Atlanta, GA, Centers for Disease Control and Prevention, 2003

Ogle RS, Maier-Katkin D, Bernard TJ: A theory of homicidal behavior among women. Criminology 33(2):173–193, 1995

O'Hara J: DA begins cross-examination of Stacey Castor. Syracuse.com, January 30, 2009a. Available at: http://www.syracuse.com/news/index.ssf/2009/01/expert_says_castors_daughter_h.html. Accessed September 29, 2017.

O'Hara J: Stacey Castor's fiancé admits lying to grand jury. Syracuse.com, January 27, 2009b. Available at: http://www.syracuse.com/news/index.ssf/2009/01/da_grills_defense_expert_in_st.html. Accessed September 29, 2017.

Reese S: The framing project: a bridging model for media research revisited. J Commun 57(1):148–154, 2007

Saltzman LE, Mercy JA, O'Carroll PW, et al: Weapon involvement and injury outcomes in family and intimate assaults. JAMA 267(22):3043–3047, 1992 1588718

Smith SG, Fowler KA, Niolon PH: Intimate partner homicide and corollary victims in 16 states: National Violent Death Reporting System, 2003–2009. Am J Public Health 104(3):461–466, 2014 24432943

Stallion KL: No less a victim: a call to Governor Nixon to grant clemency to two Missouri women. Miss Law Rev 81(1):287–307, 2016

Stöckl H, Devries K, Rotstein A, et al: The global prevalence of intimate partner homicide: a systematic review. Lancet 382(9895):859–865, 2013

van Wormer K: Reducing the risk of domestic homicide. Social Work Today 9(1):18, 2009

van Wormer K, Roberts AR: Death by Domestic Violence: Preventing the Murders and Murder-Suicides. Westport, CT, Praeger Publishing, 2008, pp 184–185

Walker LE: Battered women and learned helplessness. Victimology 2(3–4):525–534, 1977–1978

Walker LE: The Battered Woman Syndrome. New York, Springer, 1984

Walker LE: Terrifying Love: Why Battered Women Kill and How Society Responds. New York, Harper and Row, 1989

Walker LE: Battered women syndrome and self-defense. Symposium on Woman and the Law. Notre Dame Journal of Law, Ethics and Public Policy 6(2):321–334, 1992

Wilson M, Daly M: Who kills whom in spouse killings? On the exceptional sex ratio of spousal homicides in the United States. Criminology 30(2):189–215, 1992

Yourstone J, Lindholm T, Kristiansson M: Women who kill: a comparison of the psychosocial background of female and male perpetrators. Int J Law Psychiatry 31(4):374–383, 2008 18678408

3

Feticide

Richard L. Frierson, M.D.

OVERVIEW/BACKGROUND

Feticide, simply defined, is the killing of a fetus. For the purposes of this chapter, feticide will be limited to the *illegal* killing of a fetus. Currently, 38 states have fetal homicide laws, and at least 23 of these states' laws apply to the earliest stages of pregnancy—for example, "any state of gestation," "conception," or "fertilization" (National Conference of State Legislatures 2015). These early-pregnancy fetal homicide laws do not apply to legalized abortion, for which consent of the pregnant woman or a person acting on her behalf has been obtained. On a federal level, the U.S. government passed the Unborn Victims of Violence Act in 2004, which designates a fetus as a legal victim if injured or killed during the commission of any of over 60 federal crimes of violence.

Persons who commit illegal feticide can be divided into three groups: 1) pregnant women who kill their own fetus (i.e., in a manner not defined as legalized abortion), 2) men who terminate a pregnancy (outside of performing a legal abortion), and 3) women who kill another woman's fetus (outside of performing a legal abortion). Each of these groups is characterized by its own set of perpetrator characteristics and motivations. Additionally, the motivations of persons who commit feticide are, in general, vastly different from the motivations of offenders who commit neonaticide or filicide (see Chapters 4, 5, and 6).

PREGNANT WOMEN WHO COMMIT FETICIDE

Case 1: Regina McKnight

In 1999, Regina McKnight, a drug-addicted South Carolina woman, gave birth to a stillborn, 5-lb baby girl. At autopsy, the baby's gestational age was judged to be between 34 and 37 weeks, and the cause of the fetal death in utero was attributed to mild chorioamnionitis, umbilical cord inflammation (funisitis), and cocaine consumption. Despite multiple causes for the stillbirth, McKnight was arrested and charged with homicide by child abuse due to her illicit drug use. A jury found her guilty after deliberating for 15 minutes, and she received a 20-year sentence (*State v. McKnight* 2003). Her conviction was overturned for ineffective assistance of counsel after she had served 8 years. She later pleaded guilty to manslaughter to avoid a retrial and was released from prison.

In most jurisdictions, state feticide laws have been most commonly used to prosecute pregnant women for drug use during pregnancy when such drug use has resulted in the unintended death of the fetus. An example of such a prosecution is Case 1. These prosecutions have been upheld on appeal. In the words of U.S. Supreme Court Justice Anthony Kennedy, "There should be no doubt that…[a state]… can impose punishment upon an expectant mother who has so little regard for her own unborn that she risks causing him or her lifelong damage and suffering" (*Ferguson v. City of Charleston* 2001). This policy is particularly true in jurisdictions that have defined the term *child* in child endangerment statutes to include a viable fetus (Frierson and Binkley 2001). For example, on July 15, 1996, the Supreme Court of South Carolina, in an unprecedented decision, ruled 3–2 that a viable fetus is a child for purposes of South Carolina's child abuse and child endangerment statute and that a pregnant woman could be held criminally liable for actions taken during pregnancy that might harm the fetus (*Whitner v. State* 1997). Prosecutions of pregnant women for behaviors that are potentially harmful or fatal to a fetus are not without controversy. Women have been arrested for accidentally falling down the stairs, refusing a medically indicated cesarean section (C-section), delaying a C-section that then resulted in the death of one of two unborn twins, and attempting suicide that led to the death of a fetus (Marwick 2004; Paltrow and Flavin 2014). Critics have also argued that feticide laws that charge pregnant drug users may discourage drug-addicted women from obtaining prenatal care for fear they could face prosecution.

Pregnant women who *intentionally* kill their fetus through means other than legalized abortion are rare. One such case occurred in 2015 when an Indiana woman was sentenced to 20 years after being convicted of "knowingly or intentionally terminating a human pregnancy with any intention other than producing a live birth, removing a dead fetus, or performing a legal abortion" (Kaplan 2015). Prosecutors charged her with taking abortion pills obtained online in an effort to terminate her 23-week pregnancy in order to hide it from her Hindu parents. She was the first woman in the United States convicted of intentional feticide, although, ironically, she could have obtained a legal abortion and not faced prosecution. After she had served 1 year, the Indiana Court of Appeals overturned her conviction, stating that Indiana's feticide law was never intended to be used "to prosecute women for their own abortions" (Tribune News Services 2016).

Epidemiology

Between 1973 and 2005, at least 413 women have been prosecuted for actions that have been potentially harmful to a fetus (Paltrow and Flavin 2013). Since 2005, an additional 380 cases have been prosecuted (Gold and Nash 2012). The exact number of women who engage in such acts is unknown because published numbers rely on prosecution data only. The majority of feticide prosecutions have occurred in the American South, and the majority of criminal defendants have been unmarried, black, and poor. A significant number of these women were reported to law enforcement by health care providers or social workers.

Fifteen states have passed laws that require health care providers to report illicit drug use during pregnancy to law enforcement authorities (Miranda et al. 2015). An overwhelming percentage (84%) of prosecutions of pregnant women for feticide have involved cases in which pregnant women used illicit drugs, most often cocaine (68%; Paltrow and Flavin 2013). Ironically, despite early reports and research that led to concerns about an epidemic of "crack babies" who would grow up with severe disabilities, ongoing medical research has failed to show that the effects of prenatal cocaine exposure are any worse to the developing child in the long term than alcohol or other substance use (Forray and Foster 2015; Frank et al. 2001).

Motivations

By and large, women who are charged with illegal feticide did not intend to terminate their pregnancies, and most are opposed to abortion. Drug addiction, rather than a desire to harm the fetus, is the driving force behind many cases of fetal demise. Placental abruption or some other medical complication of drug use results in a pregnancy's termination. In cases of attempted suicide, the woman's primary goal is ending her own life, often with little thought that the attempt could fail but still kill her unborn child.

In the rare cases of deliberate feticide, some women have illegally terminated a pregnancy to avoid culture-based or religion-based shame and humiliation associated with sex outside of marriage. This is particularly true in some Asian and Middle Eastern cultures where unmarried, pregnant women are viewed harshly by a male-dominated society and may be subject to honor killings. Statistics from the United Nations estimates that 5,000 women a year, the majority from India and Pakistan, are the victims of honor killings, but the actual incidence is presumed to be four to five times higher (United Nations 2012). For those who are not killed, they may be forced by family members to obtain legal or illegal abortions against their will (United Nations 2014).

Unique Assessment Issues and Prevention

While many states have enacted fetal homicide laws, and 15 states require mandatory reporting of drug use during pregnancy, three states (Minnesota, South Dakota, and Wisconsin) have specific laws allowing for civil commitment of pregnant women for detoxification and substance abuse rehabilitation treatment when drug use could potentially harm the fetus (Miranda et al. 2015). In other states, when pregnant women are abusing alcohol or drugs, prevention of unintentional feticide should focus on motivational interviewing or other therapeutic techniques aimed at encouraging pregnant women who are abusing drugs to seek voluntary treatment. Additionally, in jurisdictions that attach personhood to the fetus, clinicians who assess pregnant drug users may be required to file a report with child protective services when they have reason to believe a woman in her third trimester of pregnancy has used, is using, or probably will use substances in amounts and at a frequency that has posed, or would pose, a genuine risk of physical or mental injury to the viable fetus. For single pregnant women not abusing drugs, assessment of personal, family, and cultural attitudes toward the pregnancy, especially among cultures that have punitive attitudes toward premarital intercourse, may help to identify a need for counseling regarding alternative support services, adoption, and legalized abortion services.

Finally, forensic evaluations of women who have harmed their unborn should focus on the legal concept of intent, especially in jurisdictions that allow a diminished capacity defense. Whereas a woman who illegally ingests an abortifacient (i.e., abortion-inducing drug) would clearly have specific intent to harm the fetus, a woman who has a placental abruption as a consequence of cocaine use may not. A lack of specific intent may be used to argue for a reduction in the legal charge (e.g., manslaughter rather than murder) and/or a reduced sentence.

MEN WHO COMMIT FETICIDE

Case 2: Scott Bollig

On January 14, 2014, Scott Bollig, a northwest Kansas man, purchased five pills for $60 over the Internet and picked them up at the post office a week later. On January 26, he sprinkled the contents of one of those pills on pancakes he prepared. He served them to his pregnant girlfriend, Naomi Abbott, without her knowledge that the pancakes were tainted. A few days later, she had a miscarriage. After a coworker of Naomi's told authorities that Naomi had expressed concerns that her boyfriend might be putting something in her food to terminate her pregnancy, an investigation ensued. According to a pathology report, a blood sample taken from Naomi tested positive for mifepristone, a drug that can only be administered under a doctor's supervision because of the risks of abortion associated with ingestion. Under Alexa's Law, a Kansas statute that allows prosecutors to charge someone with murder, manslaughter, or battery for intentionally harming a fetus, Bollig was subsequently indicted for murder and aggravated battery for illegally using an "abortion pancake" to terminate the pregnancy (Crimesider Staff 2014; Kansas State Code Annotated: K.S.A. 2012 Supp. 21-5419). He was convicted of a lesser charge, conspiracy to commit murder, and sentenced to 10 years (Corn 2015).

Whereas pregnant women who commit feticide (outside of legalized abortion) most commonly do so accidentally, men who commit feticide almost always do so intentionally. The exceptions are men who unintentionally cause fetal demise in a car accident or as an unintended consequence of domestic violence. There are substantial jurisdictional variations in the potential punishment that male perpetrators of feticide receive; often, punishment is dependent on the gestational age of the fetus. In order to prosecute, some states require the pregnancy to have passed the embryonic stage (8 or 12 weeks), whereas other states do not. States without feticide laws typically prosecute such men for assault on a pregnant woman. Under these laws, when a pregnant woman is attacked, prosecutors can charge the assailant with a crime against the woman and a separate crime against the unborn baby. In some death penalty states that grant personhood to the fetus, feticide can create a special aggravating circumstance under the law (killing a child under a certain age), which can qualify the defendant for a death sentence (Robinson 2017; *State v. Ard* 1998).

Epidemiology

The exact numbers of men who illegally kill a fetus against their partner's wishes are unknown. However, media reports of these cases are not uncommon and reflect myriad methods (e.g., shooting, punching, poisoning). Some men, as in Case 2, use the Internet to obtain abortion-inducing drugs, most commonly misoprostol, which they disguise in food or as another medication.

There is growing concern that in some cultures, especially in India and other Eastern societies, female feticide is a form of reproductive coercion in which husbands force pregnant wives to abort female fetuses to avoid having to pay a future dowry. In these cases, feticide (both legal and illegal abortion) is being used as a means of sex selection (Kant et al. 2015). *Female feticide*—the selective abortion of female fetuses—is killing upward of 1 million females in India annually, with far-ranging and tragic consequences. For example, in some areas of India the ratio of females to males has dropped to less than 80:100 (Ahmad 2010).

Motivations

There are several factors that can contribute to the motivations of men who commit feticide. The most common motivations include aversion to fatherhood, not wanting to maintain a relationship with the mother of the child, and avoidance of paying child support. In 2010, child support payments in the United States averaged $5,150 annually, or $430 per month (U.S. Census Bureau 2012). When inflation is controlled for, the 2017 average yearly payment would be $5,782, or $102,076 over the 18-year period from birth to age of maturity.

Female infanticide and female feticide are not uncommon in several countries: India, Bangladesh, Afghanistan, and China (de Lamo 1997). As noted earlier, economic factors play a significant role in female feticide; the prospect of having to pay a dowry to the future bridegroom of a daughter appears to be a primary motivation for female feticide in India. Although laws prohibiting the payment of dowries have been passed in India, they are largely ignored. In Indian culture, sons generally offer security to their families in old age and perform the rites for the souls of deceased parents and ancestors. Daughters, on the other hand, may be perceived as a social and economic burden.

Unique Assessment Issues and Prevention

Men who commit feticide to avoid fatherhood or to avoid child support have rarely, if ever, sought mental health treatment prior to the act. Because this type of feticide is usually a planned, predatory, and goal-directed act, there are few warning signs that foreshadow its occurrence. Consequently, prevention of this type of feticide is generally impossible unless the pregnant woman has reason to believe her spouse/partner may desire her pregnancy terminated.

The exception is the accidental killing of a fetus in cases of criminal domestic violence perpetrated against pregnant women. These feticides are often the result of affect-laden aggression. Pregnant women who are in relationships with a history of physical abuse should be asked about the spouse/paramour's attitude toward the pregnancy. For a woman in a battering relationship, the most dangerous time is when she and her partner are discussing or thinking about separation (Campbell et al. 2003). Identifying the signs that foreshadow partner abuse may be helpful for the pregnant woman. Most battered women have been told of their faults over and over by the batterer and have experienced his jealousy, possessiveness, and attempts to isolate them from friends or family members. They may need education about the impact of abuse on their physical and mental health as well as potential medical complications for their future child (Centers for Disease Control and Prevention 2008). Assisting battered pregnant women in planning exit strategies to avoid abuse, developing a safety plan, and protecting the safety of themselves and their fetus are potentially effective ways to prevent unintentional feticide resulting from domestic violence.

In regard to female feticide, in some countries laws have been passed that ban the practice and reduce the motivations behind the practice. Legalized abortion in India, for example, must be performed during a gestational period when it is difficult to identify the sex of the fetus. After 16 weeks, there must be a medical indication for the abortion (e.g., danger to the mother or child) and the concurrence of two physicians is required (Solapurkar and Sangam 1985). In 1994, India passed the Pre-Natal Diagnostic Techniques Act (PNDT), which actually prohibits the determination of the sex of the fetus at any stage of development (Subramanian and Selvaraj 2009). Under this law, no person, including the one conducting an ultrasound, may communicate the sex of the fetus to the pregnant woman or her relatives by words, signs, or any other method. Additionally, all ultrasound devices used in clinics or hospitals must be registered. However, it appears that improvement in socioeconomic circumstances and introducing legislation (such as PNDT) that is not aligned with social preferences has not improved the sex imbalance in India (Subramanian and Selvaraj 2009). Finally, although sex-selective abortion was criminalized in China in 2005, China is still expected to see very high and steadily worsening sex ratios in the reproductive age group over the next two decades (Zhu et al. 2009).

NONPREGNANT WOMEN WHO COMMIT FETICIDE

Case 3: Dynel Lane

In March 2015, Dynel Lane, a certified nursing aide, walked into a Longmont, Colorado, hospital emergency department carrying a newborn baby that had never taken a first breath. A half hour later, Michelle Wilkins was rolled into the same emergency department, bleeding from a gash across her abdomen, unaware that her 7-month-old fetus had been cut from her womb by Lane. Wilkins had responded to a Craigslist ad and went to Lane's apartment in Longmont to buy baby clothing when she was attacked by Lane, who had been faking a pregnancy for months. Lane punched Wilkins and stabbed her with a shard of broken glass. Eventually, Lane choked Wilkins until she passed out. When she awoke, she felt overwhelming pain in her stomach and "could feel my intestines outside my body." She managed to call 911.

At trial, Lane was convicted of attempted first-degree murder, two counts of first-degree assault, two counts of second-degree assault, and unlawful termination of a pregnancy (although unintentional). She received a 100-year sentence (Steffen 2016).

Fetal abduction (also known as *cesarean kidnapping*) frequently leads to the death of the fetus (or newborn), although, unlike with women who commit neonaticide, death is certainly not the intent of the abductor (see Chapter 4). Fetal abduction is a dramatic act that has been highly sensationalized in the American popular press. However, the phenomenon is not confined to the United States, as cases are also reported in Europe, Asia, South America, and Africa (Walters 2015). The largest body of information about fetal abductors has been produced by the print and television media, and very few references exist in medical literature (Arquette 2012). Academic articles have targeted law enforcement personnel and professionals working in the area of criminology (Gerberth 2006).

In many fetal abduction cases, the abductor will have faked a pregnancy and planned a method to dispose of the victim mother's body. It also appears that the majority of fetus abductors have either recently met the pregnant victim or use a confidence-style approach—befriending or conning—to gain a victim's trust (Burgess et al. 2002).

Epidemiology

Fetal abduction is an exceedingly rare event, although it appears to be on the rise, with at least 14 U.S. cases in the past decade and 4 foiled attempts (Walters 2015). Unlike in Case 3, almost all of the pregnant women die as a result of the attack, but a small majority of fetuses survive. In a study of 199 cases of *infant* abduction between 1983 and 2000, 6 (3%) were found to actually be due to C-section—that is, *fetal* abduction (Burgess et al. 2002). Since 1987, there have been at least 21 incidents worldwide of pregnant women being kidnapped and their fetuses forcibly removed via C-section (Porter 2010).

The first recorded fetal abduction in the United States occurred in Philadelphia in 1974 when Winifred Ransom killed a pregnant mother of three and used a butcher knife to remove a baby girl from the victim's womb (Arquette 2012). From this event until 2011, there were at least 22 fetal abductions or attempted fetal abductions in the United States (Rabun 2014). Unlike Case 3, in the majority of cases, the pregnant victim was killed before the C-section, either by gunshot or by strangulation. The etiology of the recent rise in fetal abductions is not known but may be attributable to increasing measures used by hospitals to prevent infant abduction. Of note, suicide attempts are common in abductors after it is discovered that the baby is not theirs (Arquette 2012).

There are several general steps involved in fetal abduction: 1) identify and contact a pregnant woman, 2) secure weapons for murder and C-section, 3) pick a location for the crime, 4) subdue and kill the mother, 5) secure the newborn through cesarean section, 6) dispose of victim's body, and 7) convince others the baby is hers (Burgess et al. 2016). Because extensive planning is involved, the perpetrator must have sufficient mental capabilities to complete all required tasks.

Motivations for Fetal Abduction

Nonpregnant women who commit feticide are generally motivated by a desperate desire to have a child—a desire so intense that they attack a pregnant woman and cut the baby from her womb and try to pass the baby off as their own. It may be viewed as an extreme form of infant abduction. Many perpetrators fake their own pregnancy prior to attempting fetal abduction and often purchase baby clothes and other items needed for a nursery. Review of kidnappings by C-section has revealed two motives: to cement a failing partner relationship or to fulfill a childbearing and delivery fantasy. In the vast majority of infant abductions, child abductors are motivated by the fantasy of having a baby. Cesarean abductors, in contrast, may have an additional fantasy of assuming the mothering identity of producing the baby (Burgess et al. 2002). It also helps to convince a husband that he fathered the infant by presenting him with a fresh newborn.

The majority of fetal abductors do not manifest symptoms of psychosis. They engage in planned, organized behaviors designed to get what they want. In one case series, the majority of abductors were of average to higher-than-average intelligence (Arquette 2012). Although fetal abduction is not strongly tied to mental illness, personality disorders may not be uncommon (Frieden 2010). Abductors do not have pseudocyesis or delusional pregnancy, rare syndromes reported frequently in developing countries (Seeman 2014). *Pseudocyesis* is a false pregnancy accompanied by abdominal enlargement, menstrual disturbances, apparent fetal movements, and other signs of pregnancy that have, in part, an endocrine basis. *Delusional pregnancy* may simply be a belief that one is pregnant without the biological changes associated with pregnancy and pseudocyesis. Pseudocyesis and delusional pregnancy occur more frequently in married women who are infertile and living in a pronatalist society (i.e., one where childbearing and parenthood are viewed as desirable for social reasons and to ensure national continuance). In contrast, fetal abductors are frequently unmarried and more likely found in developed Western societies.

Unique Assessment Issues and Prevention

Fetal abductors who come to clinical attention after an abduction require careful evaluation and a formal suicide risk assessment because there have been several abductors who have died by suicide. This population may be at unusually high risk and, rather than face the reality that they did not produce the baby, they choose to kill themselves (Burgess et al. 2002). Forensic evaluations of these women rarely reveal evidence of legal insanity—most acts are carefully planned, and killing the pregnant victim in order to get rid of a potential witness suggests knowledge of wrongfulness.

Fetal abductors are not likely to come to clinical attention prior to the abduction. The rare exception would be a person who is discovered to be faking a pregnancy. However, the overwhelming majority of women who feign a pregnancy do not become fetal abductors. In fact, simulated pregnancies are common, and there are entire websites devoted to assisting women who wish to do so (e.g., www.moonbump.com, www.fakepregnantbelly.com). Many women who are planning an adoption of a newborn infant may also consciously choose to emulate a pregnancy for privacy reasons prior to the adoption.

CONCLUSION

Feticide is a criminal act with a variety of motivations. In general, both pregnant women and nonpregnant women who commit feticide are more likely to do so unintentionally, although nonpregnant women clearly are not interested in the welfare of the woman carrying the fetus. Men, on the other hand, frequently have motivations that are clearly more nefarious. When criminal defendants who have committed feticide are being assessed, cultural factors, including the cultural attitudes about pregnancy and sex, must also be considered. Finally, forensic evaluations of persons who have committed feticide are unlikely to reveal evidence of severe and persistent mental illness.

REFERENCES

Ahmad N: Female feticide in India. Issues Law Med 26(1):13–29, 2010 20879612

Arquette KE: Fetal attraction: a descriptive study of patterns in fetal abductions. Master's thesis, Regis University, Denver, CO, 2012. Available at: https://epublications.regis.edu/cgi/viewcontent.cgi?article=1245&context=theses. Accessed November 14, 2017.

Burgess AW, Baker T, Nahirny C, et al: Newborn kidnapping by cesarean section. J Forensic Sci 47(4):827–830, 2002 12136992

Burgess AW, Dillon MA, Chiou KY, et al: Fetal abduction: comparison of two cases. J Psychosoc Nurs Ment Health Serv 54(11):37–43, 2016 27805715

Campbell JC, Webster D, Koziol-McLain J, et al: Risk factors for femicide in abusive relationships: results from a multisite case control study. Am J Public Health 93(7):1089–1097, 2003 12835191

Centers for Disease Control and Prevention: Adverse health conditions and health risk behaviors associated with intimate partner violence—United States, 2005. MMWR Morb Mortal Wkly Rep 57(5):113–117, 2008

Corn M: Bollig guilty on lighter charges. Hays Daily News, November 19, 2015. Available at: http://www.hdnews.net/74683f07-4df3-5ab1-bfcb-cc0ba42641a4.html. Accessed June 23, 2017.

Crimesider Staff: Man accused of killing fetus with "abortion pancake." CBS News, July 14, 2014. Available at: http://www.cbsnews.com/news/man-accused-of-killing-fetus-with-abortion-pancake/. Accessed October 20, 2016.

de Lamo C: The baby killers. London Times (U.K.), March 12, 1997

Ferguson v City of Charleston, 632 U.S. 67, 121 S.Ct. 1281 (2001), p 90

Forray A, Foster D: Substance use in the perinatal period. Curr Psychiatry Rep 17(11):91–102, 2015 26386836

Frank DA, Augustyn M, Knight WG, et al: Growth, development, and behavior in early childhood following prenatal cocaine exposure: a systematic review. JAMA 285(12):1613–1625, 2001 11268270

Frieden J: Fetal abductors are often not mentally ill. Clinical Psychiatry News, January 2010. Available at: https://www.questia.com/magazine/1G1-218974725/fetal-abductors-are-often-not-mentally ill. Accessed March 4, 2017.

Frierson RL, Binkley MW: Prosecution of illicit drug use during pregnancy: Crystal Ferguson v. City of Charleston. J Am Acad Psychiatry Law 29(4):469–473, 2001 11785622

Gerberth VJ: Homicides involving the theft of a fetus from a pregnant victim. Law and Order 54(3):40–46, 2006. Available at: http://www.practicalhomicide.com/Research/LOmar2006.htm. Accessed March 4, 2017.

Gold RB, Nash E: Troubling trend: more states hostile to abortion rights as middle ground shrinks. Guttmacher Institute Policy Review, Winter 2012. Available at: https://www.guttmacher.org/about/gpr/2012/03/troubling-trend-more-states-hostile-abortion-rights-middle-ground-shrinks. Accessed November 5, 2016.

Kant S, Srivastava R, Rai SK, et al: Induced abortion in villages of Ballabgarh HDSS: rates, trends, causes and determinants. Reprod Health 12:51, 2015 26021473

Kaplan S: Indiana woman jailed for "feticide." It's never happened before. The Washington Post, April 1, 2015. Available at: https://www.washingtonpost.com/ news/morning-mix/wp/2015/04/01/indiana-woman-jailed-for-feticide-its-never-happened-before/. Accessed November 5, 2016.

Marwick C: Mother accused of murder after refusing caesarean section. BMJ 328(7441):663, 2004 15206080

Miranda L, Dixon V, Reyes C: How States Handle Drug Use During Pregnancy. ProPublica, September 30, 2015. Available at: https://projects.propublica.org/ graphics/maternity-drug-policies-by-state. Accessed November 5, 2016.

National Conference of State Legislatures: Fetal Homicide State Laws, 2015. Available at: http://www.ncsl.org/research/health/fetal-homicide-state-laws.aspx. Accessed October 22, 2016.

Paltrow LM, Flavin J: Arrests of and forced interventions on pregnant women in the United States, 1973–2005: implications for women's legal status and public health. J Health Polit Policy Law 38(2):299–343, 2013 23262772

Paltrow LM, Flavin J: Pregnant, and No Civil Rights. The New York Times Opinion Pages, November 8, 2014

Porter T: Cesarean kidnapping: maternal instinct, malingering, and murder. Presented at the 2nd Global Conference Evil, Women and the Feminine Voice. Prague, Czech Republic, 2010. Available at: https://www.academia.edu/ 23182029/Cesarean_Kidnapping_Maternal_instinct_Malingering_and _Murder. Accessed June 24, 2017.

Rabun JB: For Healthcare Professionals: Guidelines on Prevention of and Response to Infant Abductions, 10th Edition. Alexandria, VA, National Center for Missing and Exploited Children, 2014. Available at: http:// www.missingkids.com/content/dam/ncmec/en_us/documents/ ForHealthCareProfessionals_10thEdition.pdf. Accessed March 4, 2017.

Robinson C: Birmingham man charged with capital murder in death of unborn baby; mom beaten with fists, belt. AL.com, January 30, 2017. Available at: http://www.al.com/news/birmingham/index.ssf/2017/01/ man_charged_with_capital_murde_4.html. Accessed February 4, 2017.

Seeman MV: Pseudocyesis, delusional pregnancy, and psychosis: The birth of a delusion. World J Clin Cases 2(8):338–344, 2014 25133144

Solapurkar ML, Sangam RN: Has the MTP act in India proven beneficial? J Fam Welf 31(3):46, 1985

State v Ard, 332 S.C. 370, 505 S.E.2d 328 (1998)

State v McKnight, 2003352 S.C. 635, 576 S.E.2d 168 (2003)

Steffen J: Judge sentences Dynel Lane to 100 years for attack. The Denver Post, April 29, 2016. Available at: http://www.denverpost.com/2016/04/29/ judge-sentences-dynel-lane-to-100-years-for-attack/. Accessed October 10, 2016.

Subramanian SV, Selvaraj S: Social analysis of sex imbalance in India: before and after the implementation of the Pre-Natal Diagnostic Techniques (PNDT) Act. J Epidemiol Community Health 63(3):245–252, 2009 19033295

Tribune News Services: Indiana court tosses woman's feticide conviction. Chicago Tribune, July 22, 2016. Available at: http://www.chicagotribune.com/news/nationworld/midwest/ct-indiana-feticide-conviction-overturned--20160722-story.html. Accessed June 23, 2017.

Unborn Victims of Violence Act, 18 U.S.C. § 1841, 10 U.S.C. § 919a (2004)

United Nations: Report of the Special Rapporteur on Violence Against Women, Its Causes and Consequences, Rashida Manjoo (A/HRC/20/16). United Nations General Assembly, 20th Session, May 23, 2012. Available at: http://www.ohchr.org/Documents/Issues/Women/A.HRC.20.16_En.pdf. Accessed June 24, 2017.

United Nations: Written Statement Submitted by International Humanist and Ethical Union, a Non-Governmental Organization in Special Consultative Status: Global Violence Against Women in the Name of "Honour." United Nations General Assembly, 25th Session, February 17, 2014. Available at: http://iheu.org/newsite/wp-content/uploads/2014/03/433_A_HRC_25_NGO_Sub_En_IHEU_Honour.pdf. Accessed November 5, 2016.

U.S. Census Bureau: Monthly child support payments average $430 per month in 2010, Census Bureau reports. U.S. Census Bureau Newsroom, June 19, 2012. Available at: https://www.census.gov/newsroom/releases/archives/children/cb12-109.html. Accessed February 4, 2017.

Walters J: Fetal abduction: brutal attacks against expectant mothers on the rise in US. The Guardian, December 2, 2015

Whitner v State, 328 S.C. 1, 492 S.E.2d 777 (S.C. 1997)

Zhu WX, Li L, Hesketh T: China's excess males, sex selective abortion, and one child policy: analysis of data from the 2005 national intercensus survey. BMJ 338:1211–1220, 2009

4

Neonaticide

Susan Hatters Friedman, M.D.

INTRODUCTION

Brooklyn teenager Tiona Rodriguez was caught shoplifting a pair of pants at the Victoria's Secret in Herald Square. Unwittingly, while inspecting the 17-year-old's bag, the store's security guard discovered a dead infant along with the pants (McKinley 2015; Rosenberg and Rosenbaum 2015; Sharp 2016). The infant had been born the previous morning. Prosecutors alleged that Rodriguez messaged a friend that she planned to "take this s–t and dig a hole, put it somewhere, LOL, then we go eat IHOP" (Saul 2018).

In 2013, when she was arrested, Rodriguez was a high school student who had no prior criminal record. She had grown up in a New York City Housing Authority complex. At various times during her teenage years, she had used injectable and implanted contraceptives.

Prosecutors asserted that Rodriguez had planned the infant's death for months. Rodriguez gave birth in a friend's bathroom, having brought along with her a bag and change of clothes. Rodriguez allegedly asphyxiated her full-term, 8-lb. baby boy; the medical examiner ruled the case a homicide. Rodriguez, according to prosecutors, had hidden at least three pregnancies. Prosecutors believed she had killed another of her infants approximately 1 year previously, after giving birth in a bathtub. She

53

and her boyfriend had discussed via text messaging how to smash the baby's body, burn it, or bury it; that infant's body "disappeared." In addition, no one had known of her earlier pregnancy at age 14, which had produced her single living child, until she went into labor (McKinley 2015; Rosenberg and Rosenbaum 2015; Sharp 2016).

Rodriguez was charged with murder in the second degree. At Riker's Island, she completed her general equivalency diploma (GED) and started college coursework. As of 2016, the 20-year-old continued to have weekend visits with her 5-year-old son, who was being raised by her mother (Sharp 2016). In early 2018, she pled guilty to first-degree manslaughter and was sentenced to a 16-year prison term (Saul 2018). As Sharp (2016) noted, "... regardless of her culpability or the callous texts she sent, Rodriguez herself was a victim of circumstance—a teenager who'd given birth three times and essentially been constantly pregnant since age 14, a child who tumbled through every possible crack before landing on Rikers."

BACKGROUND

Neonaticide refers to the murder of the infant in the first day of life. The term *neonaticide* was coined by Phillip Resnick (1970). In his early study of the world literature about children murdered by their parents, Resnick found that neonaticide differed in a great many respects from other murders of children by parents. His findings have since been corroborated by various other studies, including the early work of d'Orbán (1979).

Neonaticide is virtually always perpetrated by the mother acting alone. A recent analysis of the neonaticide literature (Friedman and Resnick 2009) found that most perpetrators of neonaticide were young women in their teens to early 20s. They were usually unmarried women who often came from disadvantaged backgrounds. Most were afraid of the consequences of their pregnancy, such as being kicked out of the house or shunned by their religious community. Their pregnancies were hidden from others with the use of baggy clothes or were even denied to themselves. Commonly, they did not obtain prenatal care.

EPIDEMIOLOGY

The true rate of neonaticides is unknown, because the pregnancies are usually hidden. Hidden pregnancies make for hidden corpses. No one knows how many infants are never discovered, as could easily have occurred in the Herald Square case. Furthermore, even when bodies are found, coroners may have difficulty determining if the baby died accidentally or by homicide. In a North Carolina study, Herman-Giddens et al. (2003) found that 2.1 per 100,000 newborns are known to have been killed or left to die. This is considered an underestimate because of the difficulty of detection.

A young woman who has just delivered her baby is far and away the most common perpetrator of neonaticide. As Friedman et al. (2012a) note, "The unwanted birth creates a much more immediate crisis for the mother than the father" (p. 785). The new mother almost always acts alone. Rarely, is the woman still in a relationship and her partner participates in the killing (Kaye et al. 1990). However, even if she is still in a relationship by the time of delivery, often her partner is unaware of the pregnancy (Amon et al. 2012). Usually, the neonaticidal woman has either experienced denial or engaged in concealment of pregnancy. Recent studies have indicated that the pregnancy ending in neonaticide is not the mother's first pregnancy in some cases (Amon et al. 2012; Putkonen et al. 2007b).

Occasional cases appear in the media in which, after discovery of an infant's death, it comes to light that the woman had committed multiple neonaticides before being apprehended. Two cases of serial neonaticides have recently made international news. Dominique Cottrez was sentenced to 9 years in prison for killing eight of her newborns. They were not discovered until more than a decade after their deaths; she had killed in the bathroom of her home near the France-Belgium border when she was in her late 20s to early 30s. The murders were only discovered after the home was sold and two infants were unearthed in the garden; another six infants were found in the garage. Cottrez told investigators the infants were born out of incest with her father; she later admitted this was untrue after testing revealed her husband to be the infants' father. She asserted that she believed her husband was aware of the babies. She had hidden her pregnancies successfully because of her obesity. Her husband and two daughters were supportive of her in court. In sentencing, according to Agence France-Presse, the magistrate noted that Cottrez had killed with "determination, awareness, organisation, and above all, coolheadedness" (Agence France-Presse in Douai 2015).

In Utah, Megan Huntsman's six dead infants were found a decade after their deaths when her estranged husband was cleaning out their old garage. She had killed the infants while in her 20s by strangulation and suffocation. Like Cottrez, Huntsman herself had living children. She was sentenced to six life terms in prison (Raab 2015).

DENIAL OF PREGNANCY VERSUS CONCEALMENT OF PREGNANCY

Neonaticides are usually preceded by denial and/or concealment of pregnancy. Three subtypes of pregnancy denial have been characterized: pervasive denial, affective denial, and psychotic denial (Friedman et al. 2007; Miller 2003).

Pervasive denial is the type most fascinating to the public and has been the subject of daytime talk shows. A woman or teenage girl with pervasive denial is totally unaware that she is pregnant. Rather extraordinarily, her body may even act as if she is not pregnant; she may continue to experience menstruation-like vaginal bleeding and may gain little to no weight, or an older woman may mistakenly believe herself to be menopausal. Labor and childbirth, then, come as a surprise. When she does go to the hospital, it may be because she is having abdominal pain and distension, or seizures from eclampsia, rather than because she knows she is pregnant and delivering (Friedman et al. 2007). If a young pregnant woman has a moderate or severe intellectual disability, it is possible that she would not equate her bodily changes and symptoms with pregnancy.

In *affective denial,* a woman is aware cognitively that she is pregnant, but she continues to behave as though she is not (Miller 2003). She may plan an abortion but be so passive and ambivalent that instead of going through with it, she hopes the pregnancy will just go away (Friedman et al. 2007). She too will not seek prenatal care, but she will likely be less surprised by labor, not thinking it to be abdominal pain.

Finally, in *psychotic denial,* a woman with schizophrenia and often a history of prior custody loss denies to herself that she is pregnant (Miller 2003). This denial may serve to ward off fears of loss of custody of her future baby. She may have intermittent periods of awareness, however, with fluctuations in her psychotic symptoms. Unlike what occurs in cases of pervasive or affective denial, it is often quite apparent to others that a woman with psychotic denial is pregnant.

In cases of *concealment of pregnancy,* a (usually young) woman is aware that she is pregnant, yet she consciously hides her pregnancy from others (Friedman and Resnick 2009). To do so, she may avoid changing in locker rooms and wear baggy clothing. She may lie to prevent others from having knowledge of her pregnancy. Concealment of pregnancy, while distinct from denial, may occur in a woman after she has stopped being able to deny the pregnancy to herself any longer but still wants to delay or avoid the consequences of others knowing about her pregnancy.

MOTIVATIONS, METHODS, AND MENTAL HEALTH

Resnick's (1969, 1970) early work elucidated that the motivation for neonaticide in the developed world was almost always because the infant was *unwanted.* His classification of motives for child murder from his original studies included the following motives for child murders with victims of all ages (described further in Chapter 6): *altruistic* (murder out of love), *acutely psychotic, unwanted child, fatal maltreatment* (originally termed "accidental"), and *partner revenge* (originally known as "spouse revenge" or "Medea syndrome"). With the exception of the unwanted child, the other motives are much rarer in neonaticide.

The murder most commonly takes place in the home, just after the birth. The location of delivery is often the location of death, wherever the woman happened to be when she went into labor. The actual method of killing the infant is often passive inaction—such as leaving the baby in the toilet to drown or outside to die from exposure (Shelton et al. 2011)— but it may also be active—using whatever potential weapon is at hand at the time of delivery—because often there is a lack of planning or preparation for the offense among those in denial. Plastic bags were the most common "weapon" in a recent study (Kaplan 2014). It may seem as though the woman who has been denying or concealing the pregnancy for months is suddenly confronted with the reality of the infant and acts on this sudden reality. However, in other cases, a woman who has concealed her pregnancy may have long planned to kill the baby, with no one else the wiser. The film *Stephanie Daley* (Brougher 2006) effectively illustrates many characteristics of neonaticide—from no one else noticing the protagonist's pregnancy, to sudden delivery alone in the bathroom on a school trip, to society's reactions.

Studies find that the woman predominantly acts alone in killing her newborn and that she is usually unpartnered (with either a troubled or nonexistent relationship with the baby's father), young, and of limited means—for example, living with her parents (Friedman and Resnick 2009; Friedman et al. 2005). She has usually either concealed or denied her pregnancy and thus has not sought prenatal care or come to medical attention. She may have difficult or poor relationships with her parents (Krüger 2015). Neonaticidal women may have spent months concerned about the ramifications of others knowing about the pregnancy, be that because of an affair, unknown paternity, premarital sex, or religious taboos (Shelton et al. 2010). Women often perceive a lack of social support and are afraid that they will lose their parents' support if it becomes known that they are pregnant or that they have a baby. They fear abandonment. Feelings of being overwhelmed and coping difficulties abound.

Passivity and indecisiveness as personality traits are seen in some neonaticide offenders and are consistent with denial. Borderline personality traits with abandonment fears may be present. Poor self-esteem, immaturity, and dependent traits may also be noted (Vellut et al. 2012). In contrast to other child murders, the woman typically will not have had a mental illness prior to her offense. The timing of neonaticide—in the first day of life—is prior to the usual onset of a postpartum psychiatric disorder, such as postpartum depression or postpartum psychosis. Suicide attempts are quite unusual in conjunction with neonaticides (Camperio Ciani and Fontanesi 2012; Friedman and Resnick 2009), in contrast to other infanticides.

Less commonly are neonaticidal women psychotic at the time of their act. In a Finnish study, four neonaticidal women who were psychotic at the time of the murders appeared to represent a unique subgroup (Putkonen et al. 2007b). These women were older and more likely to be married and have other children. They were more likely to have other living children. Additionally, they were likely to have attended prenatal care. They may represent women from the rarer *psychotic denial* of pregnancy group.

In Japan, two different types of neonaticide have been described: *anomie* and *mabiki* (Sakuta and Saito 1981). *Anomie* appears similar to neonaticide in other developed nations (as described earlier) and is more common. *Mabiki* (which translates to "thinning out" and was more common historically than in modern times) is different: an impoverished woman, or even a couple (who may have older children), acting together, kill the newborn because of the lack of resources to care for a new baby.

In developing nations, motivations for neonaticide may differ from those in the developed world. For example, in some countries, a female child is considered to be a liability, whereas a male child is desired. Both sex-selective abortions and sex-selective neonaticides occur. Not dissimilarly, neonaticide occurred in ancient civilizations. For example, in ancient Greece those infants who were weak or deformed were abandoned to the elements or even actively killed (West et al. 2009).

Evolutionary psychology offers some perspective on the concept of neonaticide, which has occurred across world cultures, dating back to the Paleolithic era (Appel 2017), as well as in various species. In the animal kingdom, as Hrdy (1979) found, infanticide may be a reproductive strategy when a youngling primate is either defective or born at the wrong time (e.g., the wrong season), thereby requiring extra work and resources in rearing. Daly and Wilson (1988) described four evolutionary rationales for infanticide, including scarce resources, a low-quality infant, uncertainty of the father's identity, and coercion by others. These rationales are also seen in human beings in developed countries but may be more apparent in countries where female infants are unwanted for economic and social reasons.

A child's "reproductive value" to the parent is lowest at birth and increases over time. In early childhood, the infant or toddler requires a lot of parental effort and expenditure yet cannot reproduce. In teenage years, arguably less parental resources are required, and the teenager can carry on the family genes. Evolutionary rationales for murder may be "adaptive," such as when there are scarce resources to raise a child (Friedman et al. 2012b). In fact, Plato discussed in *The Republic* the question of which newborns are worth the resources required to rear them (Appel 2017).

Younger mothers who kill their infant during the first day of life have significantly lower rates of mental illness compared with older mothers who kill their older children. "Rather, from an evolutionary perspective, young mothers with scarce resources are ridding themselves of an unwanted infant who may decrease their own reproductive" (and other) prospects (e.g., she is less likely to find a partner to care for another man's infant compared with finding a partner if she had no infant) (Friedman et al. 2012a, p. 786).

LEGAL ISSUES

Assessment Issues

One study of women charged with neonaticide (Spinelli 2001) found that in addition to experiencing denial of pregnancy prior to the criminal act, these women commonly reported that they had experienced dissociative symptoms around the time of birth. Dissociation and amnesia have been described in accounts by perpetrators of various serious violent crimes, but they do not exculpate the perpetrator. Selection bias and lack of malingering scales were limitations in this study of criminal defendants.

In evaluation of perpetrators of neonaticide, knowledge or suspicion of pregnancy should be queried in an open-ended fashion. The evaluator should consider whether either denial or concealment of pregnancy was present, and which subtype of denial it was. Hiding a pregnancy from others should be considered. Also, consideration of motive is critical. Diaries may yield useful information about knowledge of pregnancy (or lack thereof) and emotions. Helpful data may be gathered from the defendant and her relatives and from medical records of visits (even incidental) during the pregnancy (Friedman et al. 2012a; Shelton et al. 2011). If anxiety, depression, or posttraumatic stress disorder is present, it should be ascertained whether symptoms began before or after the murder. It should be considered whether the murder (and disposal of the baby's remains) involved planning or whether the defendant, when confronted with the reality of giving birth, killed the baby or left the baby to die. Neonaticidal women are rarely under the influence of illicit substances or alcohol at the time, although, as in any forensic evaluation, this should be asked about.

In some cases, women with *psychotic denial* of pregnancy prior to perpetrating neonaticide may be found not guilty by reason of insanity (NGRI). Others who commit neonaticide are much less likely to meet the legal criteria for insanity. They are unlikely to have a serious mental illness that either prevents them from understanding the wrongfulness of their act or, as specified in some jurisdictions, leads them to be unable to conform their conduct to the requirements of the law. Furthermore, it is important to ascertain whether the woman who committed neonaticide acted alone (as most frequently occurs) or had a co-offender. If she acted with another, the woman is even less likely to qualify for insanity because it is highly unlikely that two persons would kill a neonate for a delusional reason.

Amy Grossberg and Brian Peterson were a girlfriend and boyfriend who acted together to kill their neonate. The high school sweethearts from an upscale New Jersey suburb went off to different colleges. Grossberg wrote letters to Peterson, begging him to help her make the pregnancy go away. Although Peterson wanted to discuss the pregnancy with family or proceed with an abortion (for which the pair had the money),

Grossberg wanted the pregnancy to be secret and hoped for a miscarriage. Others had suspected Grossberg was pregnant but had never asked. Grossberg called Peterson in November of their freshman year when her water broke, and he drove to meet her in a Delaware motel room, where she gave birth. The two of them returned to their respective schools after disposing of the baby's body. The mess left in the motel room led to the discovery of an infant's corpse in a dumpster (Most 1999). The couple initially faced the death penalty; Peterson was eventually sentenced to 2 years and Grossberg to 2.5 years.

Aftermath

In jail, women may be called "baby killers" and treated badly by other inmates. Not only will other inmates have strong feelings about the murder of infants, but prison staff and mental health professionals may as well. Countertransference may be a significant issue for treating clinicians, and supervision with a colleague or mentor may be useful. Also, when interviewing these women, one may tactfully use phrases such as "when he died" rather than "when you killed him" (Friedman 2008).

Legal outcomes to neonaticide run the gamut. Whereas the United States does not currently have an infanticide law, Canada and two dozen other nations do (Friedman and Resnick 2007). These laws lessen the penalty for this type of murder, in distinction to feticide laws (discussed in Chapter 3). Several American states have considered adding such a law. Proponents of these laws may focus on whether the infant has an awareness of humanity and ensoulment. Indeed, in the Netherlands, it is legal to euthanize an unhealthy neonate (Appel 2017).

The British Infanticide Act of 1922 (amended in 1938) is the most common model for such laws. Infanticide laws were based on the concept of "lactational insanity" and the idea that "the balance of [the mother's] mind is disturbed by reason of her not having fully recovered from the effect of giving birth to the child." In contrast to being punished for murder, mothers with an infanticide verdict usually receive a significantly lesser penalty. They may have a shorter prison sentence or even community sentencing (similar to probation). However, strikingly, a causal relationship between the crime and mental illness is often not present (Friedman et al. 2012b). Consequently, while many women kill in the context of life stressors, even without a mental illness, they receive shorter sentences because the murder victim was an infant.

In America, sentencing of neonaticide offenders is highly variable. Society (and thus the jury) may feel anger and disgust or empathy and forgiveness, depending on the characteristics of the individual case. More severe charges are more likely if the infant's body was mutilated (Oberman 1996). Turmoil during birth and perceived redeemability may be considered in mitigation (Shelton et al. 2010). A U.S. Federal Bureau of Investigation study found outcomes for neonaticidal women ranging from probation to life sentences in prison. The study authors found ambivalence in sentencing, which they hypothesized could be due to the physical and emotional distress of the woman at the delivery, belief in redeemability, and the neonate's potential lack of personhood (Shelton et al. 2010). Neonaticidal women with shorter sentences were more likely to be students living with their parents, while those with longer sentences were more likely to have other children, to be married or widowed, and to be of minority ethnicity (Shelton et al. 2010). Similarly, in the United Kingdom, neonaticidal mothers were not indicted half the time, and those who were often received probation (Marks and Kumar 1993).

PREVENTION

Sex Education and Safe Environments

Because women who commit neonaticide have usually denied or concealed their pregnancy, they do not come to the attention of prenatal care providers. In many cases, potentially neonaticidal women may not be known to a health care provider for any reason until after the murder. Therefore, prevention in prenatal care clinics, although critical for many other causes of neonatal mortality, is unlikely to prevent many cases of neonaticide. Prevention must therefore take place in other ways, such as primary prevention of unwanted pregnancy through sex education and the availability of contraception (Friedman and Resnick 2009).

Teachers, parents, coaches, and workmates should keep the possibility of a hidden pregnancy in mind. Primary care physicians and pediatricians should see young women and teenage girls without their parents present if possible so that pregnancy and sex education can be discussed comfortably. They should always consider the possibility of pregnancy when females present with weight gain, nausea, or abdominal symptoms. They should also be aware that some young women seek care for stated reasons other than pregnancy when they are, in fact, pregnant and hoping that someone will ask them about it.

Preventive Strategies Around the World: Safe Havens, Anonymous Delivery, and Baby Hatches

In response to the international problem of neonaticide, nations have responded with various preventative strategies. In 1998, Mobile, Alabama, created the first American Safe Haven statute, followed the next year by the state of Texas (Cohen 2000). All 50 American states have subsequently enacted Safe Haven legislation (Friedman and Resnick 2009). Mothers are not prosecuted for relinquishing their unwanted infant in a Safe Haven (rather than leaving their baby in an unsafe place such as a dumpster or exposed to the elements). Across the United States, there are patchwork differences in the wording of legislation. In general, however, hospitals and police and fire stations are considered Safe Havens. Mothers remain anonymous after safely leaving their infants. This could potentially save the lives of infants whose mothers know about the law, are able to stealthily take their unwanted infant to an appropriate location, and make the choice to take this action rather than quietly killing their unwanted infant and disposing of the remains. Depositing a live infant in a Safe Haven location does not appear all that different to the young woman who secretly leaves her newborn on a nunnery's doorstep and rings the bell. The scenario certainly appears different from the young woman who secretly leaves her newborn in a forest to die of exposure.

There are some criticisms of the Safe Haven laws. It is important for the target demographic of young women to know about the Safe Haven laws or the option will not be chosen, and there has not been much publicity about the laws. It is not clear that the women who would otherwise commit neonaticide are the same population of women who use the Safe Haven option. A woman must be able to consider the needs of the child above her own to use the Safe Haven (Shelton et al. 2010). In addition, if a woman is pregnant and plans to use the Safe Haven option, she may see no good reason to seek prenatal care, thus increasing the medical risks to her and the unborn. Critics are also concerned with the potential effects on adoption rights and the rights of the father. However, the father frequently does not know of the pregnancy and is no longer involved in a relationship with the young woman.

At least a dozen nations currently offer either "baby hatches" (incubators where unwanted newborns can be safely left at hospitals) or "anonymous birth" (Friedman and Resnick 2009; Krüger 2015). Baby hatches are offered in several European nations (e.g., Austria, Czech Republic, Germany, Hungary, Italy, Poland, Switzerland) as well as Canada, Japan, Pakistan, the Philippines, and South Africa (Bartels 2012; Klier et al. 2013). Internationally, France has offered "anonymous birth" since the 1940s (Friedman and Resnick 2009). In general, these laws allow women to give birth safely, anonymously, and without cost in hospitals. Police-reported neonaticide rates decreased after Austria introduced anonymous delivery in 2001 (Klier et al. 2013). Among a sample of European women who committed neonaticide, 14% had considered baby hatches or anonymous delivery but did not follow through (Amon et al. 2012). Bonnet (1993) completed psychoanalytic interviews of the French women who used the free anonymous delivery option. She found that they often had experienced some period of denial of pregnancy. They fantasized about violence toward their fetus. Bonnet concluded that these women were protecting the unwanted infant from future violence or neglect (likely similar to the childhood they themselves had known) by relinquishing their motherhood and allowing their infant a chance to be loved by an adoptive mother.

CONCLUSION

In summary, in cases of neonaticide, a pattern commonly exists. It should not be considered a profile, however, because not all neonaticidal women cleanly fit the pattern. Usually, the neonaticidal woman acts covertly and alone. She is young and no longer with her partner, and she hid or disavowed her pregnancy, hoping it would just go away. She is usually free from depression or psychosis at the time of her act. The motive is most often because the baby is unwanted. Others in her life often only learn of her pregnancy after the dead infant is found. Although hidden pregnancies make prevention difficult, Safe Haven laws, baby hatches, and anonymous deliveries may help to prevent some cases of neonaticide.

REFERENCES

Agence France-Presse in Douai: French woman jailed for nine years for killing eight of her newborn babies. The Guardian, July 2, 2015

Amon S, Putkonen H, Weizmann-Henelius G, et al: Potential predictors in neonaticide: the impact of the circumstances of pregnancy. Arch Women Ment Health 15(3):167–174, 2012 22426944

Appel JM: Pediatric euthanasia, in Euthanasia and Assisted Suicide: Global Views on Choosing to End Life. Edited by Cholbi MJ. Santa Barbara, CA, Praeger, 2017, pp 351–372

Bartels L: Safe haven laws, baby hatches and anonymous hospital birth: examining infant abandonment, neonaticide and infanticide in Australia. Crim Law J 36:19–37, 2012

Bonnet C: Adoption at birth: prevention against abandonment or neonaticide. Child Abuse Negl 17(4):501–513, 1993 8402253

Brougher H (dir): Stephanie Daley (film). Venice, CA, Redbone Films, 2006

Camperio Ciani AS, Fontanesi L: Mothers who kill their offspring: testing evolutionary hypothesis in a 110-case Italian sample. Child Abuse Negl 36(6):519–527, 2012 22763357

Cohen W: Keeping the nation's newborns safe: policies to stop moms from abandoning babies. U.S. News World and Report, February 28, 2000

d'Orbán PT: Women who kill their children. Br J Psychiatry 134:560–571, 1979 476366

Daly M, Wilson M: Killing children: parental homicide in the modern West, in Homicide. New York, Aldine de Gruyter, 1988, pp 61–93

Friedman SH: After the murder: mothers who have killed. Correctional Mental Health Report 10(4):55–56, 2008

Friedman SH, Resnick PJ: Child murder by mothers: patterns and prevention. World Psychiatry 6(3):137–141, 2007 18188430

Friedman SH, Resnick PJ: Neonaticide: phenomenology and considerations for prevention. Int J Law Psychiatry 32(1):43–47, 2009 19064290

Friedman SH, Horwitz SM, Resnick PJ: Child murder by mothers: a critical analysis of the current state of knowledge and a research agenda. Am J Psychiatry 162(9):1578–1587, 2005 16135615

Friedman SH, Heneghan AM, Rosenthal MB: Characteristics of women who deny or conceal pregnancy. Psychosomatics 48(2):117–122, 2007 17329604

Friedman SH, Cavney J, Resnick PJ: Child murder by parents and evolutionary psychology. Psychiatr Clin North Am 35(4):781–795, 2012a 23107563

Friedman SH, Cavney J, Resnick PJ: Mothers who kill: evolutionary underpinnings and infanticide law. Behav Sci Law 30(5):585–597, 2012b 22961624

Herman-Giddens ME, Smith JB, Mittal M, et al: Newborns killed or left to die by a parent: a population-based study. JAMA 289(11):1425–1429, 2003 12636466

Hrdy SB: Infanticide among animals: a review, classification, and examination of the implications for the reproductive strategies of females. Ethol Sociobiol 1(1):13–40, 1979

Kaplan DS: Who are the mothers who need Safe Haven laws? An empirical investigation of mothers who kill, abandon, or safely surrender their newborns. Wisconsin Journal of Law, Gender and Society 29(3):447–511, 2014

Kaye NS, Borenstein NM, Donnelly SM: Families, murder, and insanity: a psychiatric review of paternal neonaticide. J Forensic Sci 35(1):133–139, 1990 2313254

Klier CM, Grylli C, Amon S, et al: Is the introduction of anonymous delivery associated with a reduction of high neonaticide rates in Austria? A retrospective study. BJOG 120(4):428–434, 2013 23210536

Krüger P: Prevalence and phenomenology of neonaticide in Switzerland 1980–2010: a retrospective study. Violence Vict 30(2):194–207, 2015 25929137

Marks MN, Kumar R: Infanticide in England and Wales. Med Sci Law 33(4):329–339, 1993 8264367

McKinley JC: Murder charge for Brooklyn woman whose infant was found dead in a bag. The New York Times, July 30, 2015

Miller LJ: Denial of pregnancy, in Infanticide: Psychosocial and Legal Perspectives on Mothers Who Kill. Edited by Spinelli MG. Washington, DC, American Psychiatric Publishing, 2003, pp 81–104

Most D: Always in Our Hearts: The Story of Amy Grossberg, Brian Peterson, the Pregnancy They Hid and the Baby They Killed. New York, St. Martin's True Crime, 1999

Oberman M: Mothers who kill: coming to terms with modern American infanticide. Am Crim Law Rev 34:1–110, 1996

Putkonen H, Collander J, Weizmann-Henelius G, et al: Legal outcomes of all suspected neonaticides in Finland 1980–2000. Int J Law Psychiatry 30(3):248–254, 2007a 17408742

Putkonen H, Weizmann-Henelius G, Collander J, et al: Neonaticides may be more preventable and heterogeneous than previously thought—neonaticides in Finland 1980–2000. Arch Women Ment Health 10(1):15–23, 2007b 17216371

Raab L: Utah mother gets maximum sentence for murdering six of her babies. LA Times, April 20, 2015

Resnick PJ: Child murder by parents: a psychiatric review of filicide. Am J Psychiatry 126(3):325–334, 1969 5801251

Resnick PJ: Murder of the newborn: a psychiatric review of neonaticide. Am J Psychiatry 126(10):1414–1420, 1970 5434623

Rosenberg R, Rosenbaum S: Teen indicted for murder after carrying dead baby in shopping bag. NY Post, July 30, 2015

Sakuta T, Saito S: A socio-medical study on 71 cases of infanticide in Japan. Keio J Med 30(4):155–168, 1981 7347770

Saul E: Woman found carrying her dead baby in bag gets 16 years in prison. New York Post, February 22, 2018

Sharp S: The story behind the teen mom arrested with a dead baby in her bag. Vice, Sept 29, 2016

Shelton JL, Muirhead Y, Canning KE: Ambivalence toward mothers who kill: an examination of 45 U.S. cases of maternal neonaticide. Behav Sci Law 28(6):812–831, 2010 21110394

Shelton JL, Corey T, Donaldson WH, et al: Neonaticide: a comprehensive review of investigative and pathologic aspects of 55 cases. J Fam Violence 26(4):263–276, 2011

Spinelli MG: A systematic investigation of 16 cases of neonaticide. Am J Psychiatry 158(5):811–813, 2001 11329409

Vellut N, Cook JM, Tursz A: Analysis of the relationship between neonaticide and denial of pregnancy using data from judicial files. Child Abuse Negl 36(7–8):553–563, 2012 22858094

West SG, Friedman SH, Resnick PJ: Fathers who kill their children: an analysis of the literature. J Forensic Sci 54(2):463–468, 2009 19187457

5

Fatal Maltreatment and Child Abuse Turned to Murder

Peter Ash, M.D.

INTRODUCTION

In May 2014, 5-year-old Heaven Woods of Forsyth, Georgia, about 50 miles south of Atlanta, died from blunt force trauma to her abdomen. Her death and the circumstances surrounding it were widely reported in the local media (see, e.g., Womack 2016).

Heaven's parents separated when she was 2 years old; her father, Anthony Woods, said this was because he tried to intervene when her mother, Amanda Hendrickson, was "wailing" on Heaven with her hands. He grabbed Heaven and left their home. Hendrickson later claimed the father had been abusive. Child protective service (CPS) records in West Virginia and Georgia revealed nearly a dozen reports of abuse in the 3 years between the time when Heaven's mother separated from her father and Heaven's death, all of which were not pursued or were deemed unsubstantiated.

Several weeks before Heaven's death, her mother moved in with her boyfriend, Roderick Buckner. Two days before Heaven's death, a neighbor saw Buckner, out on his porch, look around and then elbow Heaven in the stomach and knee her in the back. The next day, after seeing a similar beating, the neighbor called the state's child abuse hotline but to no avail. She later told police, "I held, I held, I held. I hung up and then I called back again, and I held and held and I just hung up," (Womack 2016). In his later plea agreement, Buckner said that he had seen Hendrickson hit Heaven, leaving bruises, and throw a shoe at her. There was evidence that the day before her death, Buckner talked to Heaven on the telephone saying he was going to "beat her ass" when he got home so that Heaven would behave and her mother would stop beating her. The next morning Heaven had trouble waking up. Medics were called, and Heaven was taken to the hospital where she died shortly after arrival.

The autopsy of Heaven revealed 10 old rib fractures, a left arm fracture, and bruises on cheeks, abdomen, both arms, both thighs, right hip, lower back, and buttocks. The coroner concluded the cause of death to be internal bleeding and blood loss from blunt force trauma to the abdomen. After Heaven's death, her mother and Buckner were arrested and charged with murder. The district attorney pursued the death penalty against both defendants. The boyfriend pled guilty and received a sentence of life without parole; Heaven's mother pled guilty and received a sentence of life with parole.

The case received widespread media attention and led to practice and policy changes at the Georgia Department of Family and Child Services, the CPS agency in Georgia.

OVERVIEW

When a child dies from child abuse or neglect, the caretaker who caused the death does not generally intend to kill the child. Rather, the death occurs as the endpoint of a history of failed care for the child or because the caretaker underestimates the severity of the physical abuse. In some cases of severe neglect or Munchausen by proxy (MBP), discussed later in this chapter, the parent may hardly be aware of significant risk to the child. The death itself is unintentional; cases in which a caretaker kills a child intentionally are covered in the chapter on child murder by parents (see Chapter 6).

Deaths from child maltreatment can be classified in a number of ways. Most typologies in the literature are based on the type of child maltreatment:

- Physical abuse
- Neglect
- Failure to provide necessary food or nutrition
- Supervisory neglect
- Medical neglect
- Sexual abuse (rare as a cause of child fatalities)
- Emotional abuse (not a direct cause of child fatalities)

Supervisory neglect occurs when a parent grossly fails to supervise a child and the child then gets into a dangerous situation, such as drowning in a bathtub, falling out of a window, or ingesting a poison.

Child abuse receives much more publicity than does neglect. However, more than 70% of children who die from child maltreatment were victims of neglect (either alone or in combination with another form of maltreatment), whereas slightly less than half suffered physical abuse (either alone or in combination with other maltreatment). Because the intention of a homicide perpetrator is crucial in determining the classification of the crime (i.e., felony murder vs. murder), juries may struggle in reaching just verdicts in these cases.

EPIDEMIOLOGY

The best U.S. data on child deaths from child maltreatment come from the National Child Abuse and Neglect Data System (NCANDS), a federally run system that collects data from all 50 states. The data in this section are from the NCANDS for federal fiscal year 2013 unless otherwise specified (Children's Bureau 2015). The federal report estimates that about 1,520 children died from child abuse and neglect, representing an annual rate of 2.0 per 100,000 children. Many believe that this estimate considerably underestimates the actual number because a large portion of deaths reported as "unintentional injury" may actually result from maltreatment. Such deaths, especially those in situations that might involve neglect, are difficult to classify (Ross and Juarez 2014).

To put the death rate of 2.0 per 100,000 in context, the rate of referrals for child maltreatment in 2013 was 471 per 100,000, and the rate that maltreatment was substantiated was 91 per 100,000. Of course, not all children who died from maltreatment had previously been reported to CPS. Although complete data are lacking, in 31 reporting states, only 11.6% of deaths were in families who had received CPS services in the previous 5 years. Other studies using smaller populations in Oklahoma (Damashek et al. 2013) and Great Britain (Reder and Duncan 1999) found somewhat higher rates of previous CPS involvement, but they still found that only a minority of children who died from maltreatment had previous CPS involvement.

Almost half (46.5%) of the reported deaths due to maltreatment were of children under 1 year of age, and almost three-quarters (73.9%) were of children under 3 years old. Although many people associate fatalities with severe physical abuse, in the NCANDS dataset, physical abuse was found in slightly less than half (46.8%) of deaths attributed to maltreatment, while neglect was present in almost three-quarters (71.4% of cases), and medical neglect (not obtaining necessary medical care) in 8.6% of cases. Deaths attributable to physical abuse typically involve fathers, whereas deaths associated with neglect more often involved mothers. Of deaths due to neglect, the vast majority were due to supervisory neglect rather than deprivation of needs (e.g., not providing a child with enough food to prevent starvation) (Welch and Bonner 2013). It is unclear what percentage of supervisory neglect reflects a single instance of lack of supervision rather than an ongoing pattern of parental inattention.

The distribution of perpetrators in the NCANDS dataset is shown in Figure 5–1.

MOTIVATIONS

Child maltreatment can stem from multiple motivations. Physical abuse may involve intentionally hurting a child out of anger or overly punitive discipline. It may also occur when a caretaker fails to recognize that his or her behavior poses a grave risk to the child, such as in some cases of shaken baby syndrome when the parent is motivated by anger or frustration. Neglect may result from a wide variety of circumstances, such as when a caretaker is unconcerned with a child's safety because of poor parenting skills or substance abuse, or when mental illness plays a role, such as when a mother withholds food because she has a delusion that the food is poisonous for her baby or when a seriously depressed mother stops eating and stops feeding her baby. No profile of a perpetrator of fatal child abuse has been identified, although many studies cite characteristics of a perpetrator as a young adult who did not finish high school, was relatively impoverished, and had poor coping skills.

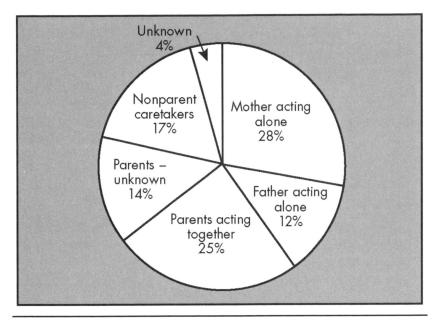

FIGURE 5–1. Perpetrators of fatal child maltreatment.

Source. Data from Children's Bureau 2015.

Munchausen by Proxy

MBP is a fairly rare form of child abuse that is different from other types of abuse. DSM-5 (American Psychiatric Association 2013) does not use the term *Munchausen by proxy* but rather lists "factitious disorder imposed by another" as a subcategory of factitious disorder. In MBP, a caretaker, most commonly the mother, creates or reports physical symptoms in the child and seeks medical attention, which may involve invasive procedures or surgery (Schreier 2004; Shaw et al. 2008). Examples of such behaviors include partially suffocating children or giving them toxins that produce respiratory symptoms, using forms of poisoning that suggest gastrointestinal disorders, giving false histories of seizures, and applying chemicals to the skin to produce rashes and other lesions. Parental motivation in MBP is often difficult to determine because parents often present as concerned for and very caring of their children and deny inflicting harm on them. The underlying motivation for causing symptoms typically stems from an intense need to form a relationship with a physician that includes elements of manipulation and wishing to receive attention.

Most MBP is perpetrated by mothers: some small-scale studies suggest that only between 7% and 15% of perpetrators are fathers (Shaw et al. 2008; Southall et al. 1997). Because MBP can involve smothering, poisoning, and other life-threatening means to create an appearance of child illness, death of the child can occur inadvertently. In a retrospective review of 39 families where MBP by suffocation was suspected and the families were covertly videotaped in the hospital (Southall et al. 1997), 33 parents were observed on film to abuse their children in the hospital. The 39 patients had a total of 41 siblings, 12 of whom had died suddenly under suspicious circumstances, and 4 of the parents later confessed to killing 8 of the siblings.

Mental Illness

An analysis of the National Institute of Mental Health Epidemiologic Catchment Area study found that of parents who reported abusing or neglecting their children, 58% met criteria for mental illness at some time in their lives (Egami et al. 1996). Antisocial personality disorder conveyed the most risk for both abuse and neglect. However, when parents with antisocial personality were dropped from the analysis, less than 5% of mentally ill parents had maltreated their children. Parents who abused alcohol were almost three times as likely both to abuse and to neglect their children as those who did not abuse alcohol. Less than 4% of parents with schizophrenia reported neglecting or abusing their children, although one review estimated that about half of parents with schizophrenia lose custody of their children (Seeman 2012). McEwan and Friedman (2016), in their review of the association between child abuse and mental illness, found that the relevant studies were difficult to interpret given varying definitions of mental illness and varying methodologies and concluded that the data suggest that most parents with mental illness are not abusive and that most abusive parents are not mentally ill. A report of an analysis of the MacArthur Violence Risk Assessment Study database found that parents with severe mental illness who had been released from inpatient hospitalization did not show an increased risk for violence toward children compared with community control subjects (Friedman and McEwan 2015).

Studies of the frequency of mental illness in parents whose children have died as a result of abuse or neglect are based on smaller samples but are consistent with studies of all maltreating parents. In a retrospective study of 49 child deaths due to abuse and neglect in Great Britain, 43% of parents had active or previous mental illness, which in almost half of the cases was substance abuse (Reder and Duncan 1999). In an analysis of the NCANDS data, perpetrators of fatal maltreatment were found to have almost the same rate of mental illness and substance abuse as perpetrators of nonfatal maltreatment, but perpetrators of fatal abuse were considerably less likely to have received mental health treatment (Douglas and Mohn 2014).

UNIQUE ASSESSMENT ISSUES

Child fatality review teams exist in every state (for details, see National Center for Fatality Review and Prevention 2018) and report through the National Child Death Review Case Reporting System. In cases in which a child dies, determining whether the death was due to abuse or to other causes is often challenging. Some of these challenges are illustrated by the death in 1996 of 7-week-old Etzel Glass. The question was whether Etzel had died from sudden infant death syndrome (SIDS) or shaken baby syndrome due to shaking by Etzel's grandmother. In SIDS, an infant dies unattended, generally while asleep, although when found, a parent may actively shake the baby in an attempt to revive him or her. In shaken baby syndrome, the parent or caretaker actively shakes an awake baby, often out of frustration or anger, and the parent or caretaker may not realize that the shaking may cause bleeding in the brain because of the brain repeatedly hitting the skull. At the grandmother's trial for the murder of Etzel, the experts for the prosecution and defense differed on the cause of death. While experts from both sides agreed that the pattern of bleeding found in the brain was somewhat atypical for shaken baby syndrome (there was no retinal bleeding and no tear of the brain stem could be located), they disagreed as to whether the bleeding was caused by being shaken while alive or should be attributed to the resuscitation efforts. The grandmother was convicted, but the Court of Appeals for the Ninth Circuit reversed the conviction, concluding there was "no evidence to permit an expert conclusion one way or the other" as to why Etzel died (*Smith v. Mitchell* 2006). The U.S. Supreme Court reversed in a 6–3 decision. The Court concluded that rather than look at the bases of the experts' opinions, deference needed to be afforded the jury's conclusion if, after viewing the evidence in the light most favorable to the prosecution, *any* rational trier of fact could have found that the expert testimony established the grandmother was guilty beyond a reasonable doubt (*Cavazos v. Smith* 2011).

Mental health professionals are seldom involved in determining the manner of death, but they may be involved in other assessments of criminal defendants charged with fatal abuse, as discussed in the next section.

AFTERMATH

If a coroner decides that a child died as the result of abuse, the state will typically charge the perpetrator with some form of murder (such as felony murder that does not require intent to kill but only intent to harm in some other way, such as child abuse) and may charge other parents or caretakers with crimes related to their allowing or encouraging abuse. The threshold question will be the intention of the alleged abuser: did the death result from an accident, negligence, intent to harm but underestimating the severity of likely injury, or intent to kill? Mental health evaluation is seldom sought to differentiate between these levels of intention—that tends to be a jury question—but it may be sought to help determine competence to stand trial, insanity, or mitigation of sentence. Mental health evaluation may also be requested to help determine whether the child should be reunited or left in the custody of the parent who may not have participated directly in the death but had been aware of previous abuse or neglect and not acted to protect the child.

There are anecdotal reports that suggest that convicted child abusers in prison are at increased risk of being assaulted by other prisoners, but the risk of their being assaulted appears lower than the well-documented risk that prison inmates who have sexually offended against children face (Fagan et al. 1996).

PREVENTION

Child abuse and neglect is a nationally recognized problem, and there are numerous federal and state agencies that implement prevention measures. Prevention strategies can be aimed at various levels: interventions that are aimed at preventing maltreatment generally, improved surveillance to identify maltreatment cases, and improved handling of cases once they are reported to CPS agencies. As noted, less than 12% of families in which a child fatality from maltreatment occurred had been reported to CPS agencies.

Reporting of suspected child abuse is mandatory in all states for psychiatrists, other physicians, psychologists, teachers, law enforcement, and some other categories (depending on state law). Nineteen states require all individuals to report suspected abuse (Child Welfare Information Gateway 2016). The assessment of children who may have been abused varies depending on the type of abuse. Allegations of neglect are typically assessed by CPS agencies, who may make home visits and will ask for additional evaluations from mental health professionals if indicated (e.g., to help determine if a parent has a mental illness that contributed to the parent's neglectful behavior). Physical abuse may be assessed through interviews of the child and medical examinations of injuries. If abuse or neglect are substantiated, evaluations by mental health experts may be solicited to help determine such issues as the amenability of parents to treatment, whether to pursue reunification, and whether a parent is fit to resume custody of his or her child.

It is beyond the scope of this chapter to review the manifold strategies that have been proposed to reduce child maltreatment generally. One recurring theme is that CPS agencies are often underfunded. High-profile cases that highlight errors by CPS, such as the case at the beginning of this chapter, often spur changes in the handling of reported cases and may be instrumental in persuading state legislatures to allocate more money for services.

In deciding whether to pursue reunification of abused children with their parents, CPS takes into account myriad factors. If maltreatment is thought likely to progress to a child's death, children are not reunited with their abusers. Child fatality review teams focus particularly on the problem of child death as a result of abuse or neglect and work to draw lessons from the case material to support prevention efforts. Recommendations from review teams include changes in public education (such as educating parents about shaken baby syndrome or risk of drowning), improvements in child welfare agency policies and practices, better CPS investigation protocols, improved risk assessments, training of professionals, and legal changes (Douglas and Cunningham 2008). In a review of child fatality team activities, Palusci and Covington (2014) found that over 70% of deaths had been deemed preventable by the examining child fatality team. In reviews of more than 2,000 deaths, the teams implemented more than 100 strategies after review.

CONCLUSION

Fatal child maltreatment more often flows from neglect than from physical abuse—and is very difficult to predict. Prior to a child dying, perpetrators of fatal maltreatment cannot be reliably distinguished from perpetrators of nonfatal abuse and neglect. Assessing whether a child's death was due to accident, natural causes, negligence, abuse without intent to kill, or intentional homicide is often a challenge, particularly in cases involving babies without a history of CPS involvement. Because in only a small minority of deaths had there been prior CPS involvement, interventions that have community-wide impact to prevent child maltreatment are most likely to reduce maltreatment deaths. Limited funding for CPS agencies and home interventions remains a challenge in many jurisdictions.

REFERENCES

American Psychiatric Association: Diagnostic and Statistical Manual of Mental Disorders, 5th Edition. Arlington, VA, American Psychiatric Association, 2013

Cavazos v Smith, 566 U.S. __ (2011)

Child Welfare Information Gateway: Mandatory reporters of child abuse and neglect. Washington, DC, U.S. Department of Health and Human Services, Children's Bureau, 2016

Children's Bureau: Child Maltreatment 2013. Washington, DC, U.S. Department of Health and Human Services, Administration for Children and Families, Administration on Children, Youth and Families, 2015. Available at:https://www.acf.hhs.gov/sites/default/files/cb/cm2013.pdf. Accessed August 10, 2017.

Damashek A, Nelson MM, Bonner BL: Fatal child maltreatment: characteristics of deaths from physical abuse versus neglect. Child Abuse Negl 37(10):735–744, 2013 23768940

Douglas EM, Cunningham JM: Recommendations from child fatality review teams: results of a US nationwide exploratory study concerning maltreatment fatalities and social service delivery. Child Abuse Rev 17(5):331–351, 2008

Douglas EM, Mohn BL: Fatal and non-fatal child maltreatment in the US: an analysis of child, caregiver, and service utilization with the National Child Abuse and Neglect Data Set. Child Abuse Negl 38(1):42–51, 2014 24268379

Egami Y, Ford DE, Greenfield SF, et al: Psychiatric profile and sociodemographic characteristics of adults who report physically abusing or neglecting children. Am J Psychiatry 153(7):921–928, 1996 8659615

Fagan TJ, Wennerstrom D, Miller J: Sexual assault of male inmates: prevention, identification, and intervention. J Correct Health Care 3(1):49–65, 1996

Friedman SH, McEwan MV: Risk assessments for violence by parents towards children. Presented at the American Academy of Psychiatry and the Law Annual Meeting, Ft. Lauderdale, FL, October 2015

McEwan M, Friedman SH: Violence by parents against their children: reporting of maltreatment suspicions, child protection, and risk in mental illness. Psychiatr Clin North Am 39(4):691–700, 2016 27836161

National Center for Fatality Review and Prevention (Web site), 2018. Available at: https://www.ncfrp.org. Accessed May 15, 2018.

Palusci VJ, Covington TM: Child maltreatment deaths in the U.S. National Child Death Review Case Reporting System. Child Abuse Negl 38(1):25–36, 2014 24094272

Reder P, Duncan S: Lost Innocents: A Follow-Up Study of Fatal Child Abuse. New York, Routledge, 1999

Ross AH, Juarez CA: A brief history of fatal child maltreatment and neglect. Forensic Sci Med Pathol 10(3):413–422, 2014 24464796

Schreier H: Munchausen by proxy. Curr Probl Pediatr Adolesc Health Care 34(3):126–143, 2004 15039661

Seeman MV: Intervention to prevent child custody loss in mothers with schizophrenia. Schizophr Res Treatment 2012:796763, 2012 22966446

Shaw RJ, Dayal S, Hartman JK, et al: Factitious disorder by proxy: pediatric condition falsification. Harv Rev Psychiatry 16(4):215–224, 2008 18661364

Southall DP, Plunkett MC, Banks MW, et al: Covert video recordings of life-threatening child abuse: lessons for child protection. Pediatrics 100(5):735–760, 1997 9346973

Smith v Mitchell, 437 F. 3d 884, 890 (2006)

Welch GL, Bonner BL: Fatal child neglect: characteristics, causation, and strategies for prevention. Child Abuse Negl 37(10):745–752, 2013 23876861

Womack AL: Did Heaven have to die? Case file details slain Forsyth 5-year-old's torment, system's shortcomings. The Telegraph, Macon, GA, April 2, 2016. Available at: http://www.macon.com/news/local/crime/article69599202.html. Accessed March 15, 2017.

6

Child Murder by Parents

Phillip J. Resnick, M.D.

INTRODUCTION

On June 20, 2001, Andrea Yates drowned her five children, ages 6 months to 7 years, in her bathtub. She was charged with multiple counts of first-degree murder with death penalty specifications. Yet, Andrea Yates's earlier life provides no clues that she would later commit an infamous crime. She graduated valedictorian of her high school class of 608 students. Upon completion of her bachelor's degree in nursing, she became a highly regarded nurse at the MD Anderson Cancer Center in Houston. After her marriage, she was determined to be a "super mom." Every witness at her trial agreed that she was a wonderful mother.

After her fourth son was born, Mrs. Yates felt overwhelmed and depressed. She knew through a "feeling" that Satan wanted her to kill her children. She took an overdose of medication to take her own life rather than risk harming her children. Against the medical advice from her treating psychiatrist, she and her husband chose to have a fifth child.

The last of Mrs. Yates's four psychiatric hospitalizations took place 5 weeks before the homicides. Mrs. Yates did not reveal that she had psychotic symptoms to either her husband or her doctor. She thought that television commercials were referring directly to her. She had a delusional belief that television cameras were placed throughout her home to monitor the quality of her mothering. Finally, she had the belief that the "one and only Satan" was literally within her.

Mrs. Yates believed her children were not developing "intellectually" and "were not righteous." She believed her children would "never be right" because she had "ruined them" with her defective mothering. For example, she thought that her son Luke would become a "mute homosexual prostitute" and that her son John would become a "serial murderer." She was convinced that all her children would be punished and "burn in hell." She thought that after she drowned her children she would be arrested and executed and that Satan would be executed along with her. According to her delusional system, drowning her children would "save their souls." She was doing what was right by arranging for them to be in heaven while they were still "innocent."

Mrs. Yates's attorneys entered a plea of not guilty by reason of insanity in her first trial in 2002. The jury rejected the insanity defense, and she was sentenced to life in prison. Her first trial verdict was overturned by an appellate court. In her second trial in 2006, the jury found her not guilty by reason of insanity (Resnick 2007).

BACKGROUND

Most people find child homicide by parents (*filicide*) to be one of the most disturbing types of crime. It is even more distressing when a mother kills her child, because society expects her, but not the father, to be selfless and to love and protect her children at all costs (Pagelow 1984). Mothers are supposed to be "guided by natural feminine instincts that can infer an angelic temperament, make them clairvoyant about their children's needs, and willing to place their own desires second to those of their family" (Barnett 2006, p. 412). An article in *Newsweek,* for example, asked, "How can a mother [Yates] commit such a crime against nature and all morality and end the lives she has so recently borne and nurtured?" (Johnson et al. 2001, p. 20). This question is among those this chapter seeks to answer.

Throughout history and myth, women who kill their children have been considered monsters. The Puritans believed, "All women who killed their babies, violated what was taken to be the law of nature decreed by God.... The women who killed their children, then, they were by definition unnatural and monstrous—more hardened than the sea monsters, who draw out their breasts, and give suck to their young ones" (Jones 1980, p. 78).

The media sometimes characterize mothers who kill their children as either "mad" or "bad":

> Women portrayed as "mad" have been characterized as morally "pure" women who by all accounts have conformed to traditional gender roles and notions of femininity. These women are often viewed as "good mothers," and their crimes are considered irrational, uncontrollable acts, usually the direct result of mental illness. In contrast, women characterized as "bad" are…depicted as cold, calloused, evil mothers who have often been neglectful of their children…. (Meyer et al. 2001, p. 70)

The quintessentially "bad" child killer is Susan Smith, a South Carolina woman who purposefully sent her car containing her two sons into a lake with an alleged motive related to a romantic relationship. An Australian headline said she committed "the mother of all crimes" (Wilczynski 1997). The media relentlessly portrayed her as bad even though the jury voted to spare her life.

In contrast, fathers who kill their children evoke much less emotion because they are not expected to have the same unconditional love that mothers have for their children.

EPIDEMIOLOGY

The United States has the highest rate of child murder among developed nations. The most common perpetrator of child homicide is a parent. In infancy, the U.S. rate of homicide is 8 per 100,000, several times higher than the rate in Canada (2.9 per 100,000) (Friedman et al. 2012). About 2.5% of all homicide arrests in the United States are parents who have killed their children (Mariano et al. 2014). This amounts to an average of about 500 filicide arrests each year. The rates of child homicide decrease with the child's age. At a visceral level, the horror of filicide seems to grow as the victim's age increases (Oberman 1996).

Ninety percent of filicide perpetrators are biological parents, and 10% are stepparents. However, stepparents are far more likely to kill children than biological parents. Among "child maltreatment" homicides, fatal child abuse in stepparents is up to 100 times higher (Daly and Wilson 1994).

The strongest predictive factors of maternal child homicide are maternal age of 19 years or younger, education of 12 years or less, single marital status, and late or absent prenatal care (Overpeck et al. 1998). Men, as opposed to women, who kill their children are more likely to kill older children, to be unemployed, to be facing separation from their spouse, and to abuse alcohol or drugs (Marleau et al. 1999; West et al. 2009). Among 16- to 18-year-old victims, fathers commit 80% of the homicides (Kunz and Bahr 1996). Fathers are more likely to kill when there is doubt about paternity and when the child is viewed as an impediment to their career (Resnick 1969). Men rarely kill their own children; instead, they more often kill the children of their predecessors (Kaplun and Reich 1976).

METHODS OF FILICIDE

The most common methods of infanticide are battering, smothering, strangling, and drowning (Lewis and Resnick 1999). The method of killing is related to the age of the victim (Adinkrah 2001). Homicide of infants and young children is typically committed with personal weapons (e.g., hands, feet) and rarely involves firearms or knives. Conversely, older children are killed with knives, firearms, and other lethal weapons. Fathers tend to use more violent methods, such as striking, squeezing, or stabbing, whereas mothers more often drown, suffocate, or gas their victims (Marleau et al. 1999; Resnick 1969).

MOTIVATION FOR CHILD MURDER BY PARENTS

To provide a framework for understanding motivations for filicide, we can divide child homicides into five categories (Resnick 1969). This classification is based on explanations given by the parent.

Altruistic Filicide

Altruistic filicides are committed "out of love" rather than anger or hate. Two subgroups exist: filicide associated with suicide and filicide to relieve or prevent suffering.

Filicide Associated With Suicide

Parents who commit filicide associated with suicide make a decision to take their own life first. Mothers may then feel that they cannot abandon their children and leave them "motherless" in what they perceive as a cruel world. Suicidal mothers sometimes see their children as an extension of themselves. They may believe their children suffer the same misery as they do. One mother left a suicide note saying simply, "Bury us in one box. We belong together you know" (Tuteur and Glotzer 1959). About a third of mothers who kill their children take their own lives. Fathers are almost twice as likely to complete suicide after filicide (Friedman et al. 2005a), although this difference may be not because mothers attempt suicide less often but because men are much more likely to complete their suicide using more lethal methods. Men are also much more likely to commit *familicide*—that is, killing their wives and children before taking their own lives (see Chapter 10).

On October 25, 1994, Susan Smith reported to police that her two sons (ages 14 months and 3 years) had been kidnapped by a black carjacker (Carroll and O'Shea 1995; Meyer et al. 2001). After 9 days of searching by law enforcement, she revealed she had rolled her car into a lake with her sons strapped into their car seats. She said she had planned to drown herself with them but changed her mind at the last moment. She had been rejected that day by a man she loved. If her account is taken at face value, her filicide would be an altruistic "extended suicide." According to the prosecution theory, her motive was that of "unwanted child" filicide; she wished to rid herself of her children to increase her chances of having a relationship with a man who did not want to marry a woman burdened with children. The jury spared her life but sentenced her to life in prison.

Filicide to Relieve or Prevent Suffering

These parents kill to relieve the child victim's suffering, which may be real or imagined. If the suffering is real, the killing could be characterized as euthanasia. Much more often, the filicide is based on a delusional perception that a child is suffering or at risk of going to hell. For example, some mothers have believed their children were going to be taken into "white slavery" (Morton 1934) or abducted by a child pornography ring. Others believe their children were about to be tortured or were possessed by Satan (Holden et al. 1996). Andrea Yates's motive for her filicides was to ensure that her children would not go to hell. Thus, her filicides fit this category of trying to prevent an eternity of suffering.

Acutely Psychotic Filicide

This designation applies to psychotic parents who kill with no comprehensible motive. It includes patients who kill under the influence of command hallucinations, epilepsy, or delirium. Hopwood (1927) reported one case of an epileptic mother who placed her baby on the fire and the kettle in her cradle. In a recent case, an epileptic woman in Sacramento placed her infant in a microwave oven during a period of postictal confusion (Smith 2015).

Unwanted Child Filicide

Unwanted child murders are committed because a child is no longer wanted. This is the most common motive for killing newborns (see Chapter 4). A 25-year-old widow with borderline intelligence was offered a marriage proposal, but only if she parted with her two children. After being refused placement by social agencies, she decided to dispose of them by cutting them up with a hatchet and then burning them with gasoline.

Child Maltreatment Filicide

Child maltreatment homicides usually result from a fatal "battered child syndrome" (Kempe et al. 1962). The violent outbursts often occur in the overzealous application of discipline. Persistent crying is a common precipitant (Kadushin and Martin 1981). This is the only one of the five filicide categories in which the death is not intended by the parent (see Chapter 5).

Spouse Revenge Filicide

This final category consists of parents who kill their offspring in a deliberate attempt to make their spouses or ex-spouses suffer. The mythical prototype is found in Euripides' play *Medea*. After killing their two sons, Medea told her unfaithful husband, Jason, "Thy sons are dead and gone. That will stab thy heart" (Oates and O'Neill 1938). The most common precipitants for spouse revenge filicide are spousal infidelity and child custody disputes.

In a notable case from Indianapolis, Ronald Shanabarger's fiancée had made arrangements to go on a Caribbean cruise with her girlfriends before their engagement. When Mr. Shanabarger's father died, his fiancée declined to return early from the cruise to be with him in his time of grief. He resolved in his rage to make her suffer the way he had suffered. He waited until they married and their son, Tyler, was 7 months old. After his wife was fully bonded with Tyler, he killed their child (Associated Press 1999). He was sentenced to 49 years in prison.

AFTERMATH

Parents who kill their children experience multiple losses, including their children, their freedom, and often their spouse (Thomas et al. 1994). These life events are likely to prolong the parent's depression. The anniversary of the children's deaths and exposure to things that remind the parent of it are likely to be upsetting. The act of child murder itself is highly traumatic and sometimes causes symptoms of posttraumatic stress disorder in the perpetrator (Harry and Resnick 1986; Rynearson 1984). Parents who kill their children often find it harder to forgive themselves than society does. They sometimes blame themselves for failing to seek help earlier. They may seek punishment for the rest of their lives and remain a serious suicide risk.

SPOUSES' REACTION TO FILICIDE

Although some partners do forgive their spouse for a psychotically motivated filicide, few continue to live with their spouse. They may feel they could never trust their spouse alone with additional children. Susan Smith's separated husband testified in favor of her receiving the death penalty. Andrea Yates's husband, Rusty, was supportive of her through the end of her first trial, but he then divorced her and went on to marry another woman. Occasionally, a spouse will remain married and the couple may even have another child together.

ROLE OF POSTPARTUM DEPRESSION AND PSYCHOSIS IN FILICIDE

Women are more likely to experience psychiatric illness after childbirth than at any other time in their life (Kendell et al. 1987). In the month following childbirth, women are up to 25 times more likely to become psychotic (Marks 1996). Postpartum depression affects between 10% and 22% of adult women before the infant's first birthday (Stowe et al. 2001). Psychosis occurs in postpartum women at a rate of about 1 case per 1,000 births (Terp and Mortensen 1998) and usually involves symptoms of hallucinations and delusions. Confusion and delirium are also common (Hickman and LeVine 1992). Onset is usually within days to 2 months of childbirth (Hay 2009). Because untreated postpartum psychosis has an estimated 4% risk of infanticide (murder of the infant in the first year of life) (Altshuler et al. 1998) and a 5% risk of suicide (Knops 1993), psychiatric hospitalization usually is required to protect the mother and her baby.

Nearly three-fourths (>72%) of mothers with postpartum psychosis have bipolar disorder or schizoaffective disorder, whereas 12% have schizophrenia (Sit et al. 2006). Some authors consider postpartum psychosis to be due to bipolar disorder until proven otherwise. Mothers with a history of bipolar disorder or postpartum psychosis have a 100-fold increase in rates of psychiatric hospitalization in the postpartum period (Attia et al. 1999).

Fifty percent or more of women who had a previous episode of postpartum depression experienced relapse after a subsequent pregnancy (Gold 2001). The relapse rate for postpartum psychosis is close to 80% (Altshuler et al. 1998; Cohen and Altshuler 1997; Nonacs and Cohen 1998; Stowe et al. 2001). Prophylactic treatment with antidepressants is often successful in reducing the recurrence of postpartum depression.

In a study of women with postpartum major depression (Wisner et al. 1999), 57% reported obsessional thoughts concerning harm to their babies, and the majority had checking compulsions (i.e., checking that they had not harmed their babies, that nothing terrible had happened). Obsessional thoughts are typically experienced, not so much as an impulse to harm the child but as an apprehension that such an impulse might occur (Button and Reivich 1972). Ego-dystonic obsessional thoughts are unlikely to be acted on (Booth et al. 2014). The type of obsessional concerns about infanticide that are most likely to be acted on are preoccupation with feelings of maternal inadequacy and obsessional fears about the child's well-being (McDermaid and Winkler 1955).

Mothers who have delusions that their baby is a devil, ill fated, or someone else's baby are most likely to have significant abusive incidents toward the baby (Chandra et al. 2002). Stanton et al. (2000) found that psychotic mothers who attempted suicide often killed suddenly without much planning, whereas depressed mothers had contemplated killing their children for days to weeks prior to their crimes.

Approximately one-quarter of the women referred for psychiatric services have a child under 5 years of age (Mowbray et al. 2001.) Jennings et al. (1999) reported that 41% of depressed mothers of infants and toddlers had thoughts of harming their child. Mothers with postpartum depression are reluctant to share their emotional upset because they do not want others to think of them as a "bad mother." Mothers are especially uneasy sharing filicidal thoughts with social workers because they fear that their children will be taken away. Some mothers exaggerate their suicidality to receive inpatient care so they can be protected from killing their children (Barr and Beck 2008).

LEGAL DISPOSITION OF FILICIDE OFFENDERS

There is great disparity in the sentences given to parents convicted of killing their children (Oberman 1996). Society simultaneously expresses moral outrage at the offense, yet often treats offenders, especially mothers, with lenience (Oberman 1996). The average sentence for women convicted of filicide in the United States was 17 years (Shelton et al. 2010). Fathers are likely to receive much longer sentences than mothers who kill their children (Resnick 1969; West et al. 2009). Fathers are also more likely to be sentenced to execution than are mothers.

No crime is more likely to succeed with an insanity defense than a mother who has killed her children (Perlin 1994). The filicide categories that are more likely to succeed with an insanity defense are the "altruistic" filicides and the "acutely psychotic" filicides. Immediately after altruistic and acutely psychotic filicides, the perpetrators usually run to seek help, confess, and make no attempt to conceal their crime (Resnick 1969). By contrast, the "unwanted child" and "child maltreatment" filicide perpetrators often go to great lengths to hide incriminating evidence.

Many women who succeed with an insanity defense had planned a filicide-suicide but were unsuccessful in killing themselves after killing their child (42%). Most (69%) had auditory hallucinations, and 74% were delusional (Friedman et al. 2005b). Psychotic states that predispose to successful insanity defenses include beliefs that the killing must be done for some noble purpose, such as the salvation of the infant or the salvation of the world (Hickman and LeVine 1992). Severe depression, even without psychotic features, may distort a filicidal parent's thinking so that the parent believes that his or her children would be better off in heaven with him or her. In these extended suicides, it is usually clear that the parent knew the nature and quality of the act and that the killing was legally wrong. However, the parent often believes he or she is doing what is morally right for his or her child. In some jurisdictions, this is sufficient to meet the insanity standard.

A typical prosecution argument against an insanity defense is that the defendant became angry at the infant because of the demanding requirements of infant care, such as coping with persistent crying (Hickman and LeVine 1992). The argument suggests that the parent lost his or her temper and attacked the infant. In effect, the argument is an effort of the prosecution to portray an infanticide as an example of extreme child abuse. Even though mothers are more likely to succeed with an insanity defense than fathers, the vast majority of women who kill their children are found guilty and sent to prison, possibly because even a psychotically depressed parent who kills their child usually kills with premeditation and carries out the homicide in a logical, methodical manner (Brockington 1995). In one study of 20 women who raised postpartum depression or psychosis as an insanity defense, one-half were found not guilty by reason of insanity, one-quarter received heavy sentences, and one-quarter received light sentences (Cox 1988).

PREVENTION

Parenting capacity should be routinely considered in evaluating psychiatric patients. Certainly, when children are present for a portion of a psychiatric visit, the clinician can observe the appropriateness of the parent-child interaction. Parents should also be assessed for their potential to harm their children (Hatters Friedman and Resnick 2009). Early screening and identification of mental illness during pregnancy and the postpartum period is important. The Edinburgh Postnatal Depression Scale (Cox et al. 1987; Ryan et al. 2005) is a validated tool that can be easily administered both during pregnancy and postpartum.

The clinician should be alert to the filicidal potential of all depressed parents, particularly mothers considering suicide. Forty-one percent of depressed mothers with children under 3 years of age, compared with 7% of control mothers, admitted to thoughts of harming their infant (Jennings et al. 1999). A pediatric study of mothers found that 70% of mothers with colicky infants experienced explicit aggressive thoughts toward their infants, and over a quarter (26%) of them had infanticidal thoughts during colic episodes (Levitzky and Cooper 2000).

When mothers of young children commit suicide, about 5% also kill at least one of their children (Appleby 1996). In evaluating depressed, suicidal mothers who have children younger than 5 years at home, clinicians should ask what plans the mother would have for her children if she were to take her own life. Some mothers will say that their husband is quite able to look after the children. Others will say that they would take their children to heaven with them.

Parents can also be asked about thoughts and fears of harming their children (Friedman and Resnick 2006; Friedman et al. 2008). If a mother acknowledges thoughts of harming a child, the clinician should determine the frequency and intensity of such thoughts and whether the mother thinks that she might actually carry them out (Jennings et al. 1999). The clinician should also assess whether these thoughts and fears are due to obsessive-compulsive disorder, depression, or psychosis. Although mothers with obsessive-compulsive disorder may experience thoughts of harming their baby, these thoughts are ego-dystonic and more related to fears than plans.

A thorough evaluation for psychiatric hospitalization should be completed for mentally ill mothers of young children because of the possibility of multiple deaths from a filicide-suicide. Factors that potentially merit psychiatric hospitalization include maternal fears of harming their children, delusions of their child's suffering, and improbable concerns about their child's health (Guileyardo et al. 1999). Decisions concerning the hospitalization of a father should involve careful questioning about suicide, extended suicidal plans, and paranoid symptoms centered on the family (Marleau et al. 1999).

Spouse revenge filicide is difficult to prevent because there is usually little warning. However, in bitter child custody disputes, some warning signs may appear. Evaluators in child custody disputes should be alert to situations in which a mother is so convinced that her child will be sexually abused if custody is awarded to her ex-husband that she decides that the child is better off in heaven (Hatters Friedman et al. 2005). Other parents believe that if they cannot have their children, they will make sure that their ex-spouse does not have them either.

CONCLUSION

The death of a child is always tragic. When children are killed by one of their own parents, it is frequently viewed as the ultimate betrayal, because the parent's role is to nurture and protect his or her children. On the other hand, one of the most traumatic events any parent can experience is to have a child predecease them for any reason. When a child's death is the result of a parent's psychosis, the feelings of loss and guilt usually last a lifetime. Some parents who have killed their children find it hard to forgive themselves and are indifferent to whether they are placed in prison or a hospital. The ongoing sorrow of these parents is captured in the words of Medea (Hamilton 1942, p. 178) upon killing her two sons:

> To die by other hands more merciless than mine.
> No; I who gave them life will give them death.
> Oh, now no cowardice, no thought how young they are,
> How dear they are, how when they first were born—
> Not that—I will forget they are my sons.
> One moment, one short moment—then forever sorrow.

REFERENCES

Adinkrah M: When parents kill: an analysis of filicides in Fiji. Int J Offender Ther Comp Criminol 45(2):144–158, 2001

Altshuler LL, Hendrick V, Cohen LS: Course of mood and anxiety disorders during pregnancy and the postpartum period. J Clin Psychiatry 59 (suppl 2):29–33, 1998 9559757

Appleby L: Suicidal behaviour in childbearing women. Int Rev Psychiatry 8(1):107–115, 1996

Associated Press: Man killed son to spite wife, prosecutors say. The New York Times, June 29, 1999. Available at: http://www.nytimes.com/1999/06/29/us/man-killed-son-to-spite-wife-prosecutors-say.html. Accessed June 2018.

Attia E, Downey J, Oberman M: Postpartum psychoses, in Postpartum Mood Disorders. Edited by Miller LJ. Washington, DC, American Psychiatric Publishing, 1999, pp 99–117

Barr JA, Beck CT: Infanticide secrets: qualitative study on postpartum depression. Can Fam Physician 54(12):1716–1717, 2008 19074717

Barnett B: Medea in the media: narrative and myth in newspaper coverage of women who kill their children. Journalism 7(4):411–432, 2006

Booth BD, Friedman SH, Curry S, et al: Obsessions of child murder: underrecognized manifestations of obsessive-compulsive disorder. J Am Acad Psychiatry Law 42(1):66–74, 2014 24618521

Brockington IF: Motherhood and Mental Health. Oxford, United Kingdom, Oxford University Press, 1995

Button JH, Reivich RS: Obsessions of infanticide. A review of 42 cases. Arch Gen Psychiatry 27(2):235–240, 1972 4402897

Carroll GP, O'Shea M: Will they kill Susan Smith? Newsweek, July 31, 1995. Available at: http://www.newsweek.com/id/120883. Accessed September 1, 2016.

Chandra PS, Venkatasubramanian G, Thomas T: Infanticidal ideas and infanticidal behavior in Indian women with severe postpartum psychiatric disorders. J Nerv Ment Dis 190(7):457–461, 2002 12142847

Cohen LS, Altshuler LL: Pharmacologic management of psychiatric illness during pregnancy and the postpartum period, in Psychiatric Clinics of North America Annual of Drug Therapy. Edited by Dunner DL, Rosenbaum, JF. Philadelphia, WB Saunders, 1997, pp 21–61

Cox JL, Holden JM, Sagovsky R: Detection of postnatal depression. Development of the 10-item Edinburgh Postnatal Depression Scale. Br J Psychiatry 150(6):782–786, 1987 3651732

Cox JL: Postpartum defense: no sure thing. National Law Journal, December 5, 1988, p 3

Daly M, Wilson MI: Some differential attributes of lethal assaults on small children by stepfathers versus genetic fathers. Etiol Sociobiol 15(4):207–217, 1994

Friedman SH, Resnick PJ: Mothers thinking of murder: considerations for prevention. Psychiatr Times 23(10):9–10, 2006

Friedman SH, Horwitz SM, Resnick PJ: Child murder by mothers: a critical analysis of the current state of knowledge and a research agenda. Am J Psychiatry 162(9):1578–1587, 2005a 16135615

Friedman SH, Hrouda DR, Holden CE, et al: Child murder committed by severely mentally ill mothers: an examination of mothers found not guilty by reason of insanity:2005 Honorable Mention/Richard Rosner Award for the best paper by a fellow in forensic psychiatry or forensic psychology. J Forensic Sci 50(6):1466–1471, 2005b 16382847

Friedman SH, Sorrentino RM, Stankowski JE, et al: Psychiatrists' knowledge about maternal filicidal thoughts. Compr Psychiatry 49(1):106–110, 2008 18063049

Friedman SH, Cavney J, Resnick PJ: Child murder by parents and evolutionary psychology. Psychiatr Clin North Am 35(4):781–796, 2012

Gold LH: Clinical and forensic aspects of postpartum disorders. J Am Acad Psychiatry Law 29(3):344–347, 2001 11592465

Guileyardo JM, Prahlow JA, Barnard JJ: Familial filicide and filicide classification. Am J Forensic Med Pathol 20(3):286–292, 1999 10507800

Hamilton E (ed): The quest of the golden fleece, in Mythology. Boston, MA, Little, Brown, 1942, p 178

Harry B, Resnick PJ: Posttraumatic stress disorder in murderers. J Forensic Sci 31(2):609–613, 1986 3711837

Hatters Friedman S, Resnick PJ: Parents who kill: why they do it. Psychiatr Times 26(5):10–12, 2009

Hatters Friedman S, Hrouda DR, Holden CE, et al: Filicide-suicide: common factors in parents who kill their children and themselves. J Am Acad Psychiatry Law 33(4):496–504, 2005 16394226

Hay PJ: Post-partum psychosis: which women are at highest risk? PLoS Med 6(2):e27, 2009 19209954

Hickman SA, LeVine DL: Postpartum disorders and the law, in Postpartum Psychiatric Illness: A Picture Puzzle. Edited by Hamilton JA, Harberger PN. Philadelphia, PA, University of Pennsylvania Press, 1992

Holden CE, Burland AS, Lemmen CA: Insanity and filicide: women who murder their children. New Dir Ment Health Serv 69(69):25–34, 1996 8935820

Hopwood JS: Child murder and insanity. J Ment Sci 73:98–108, 1927

Jennings KD, Ross S, Popper S, Elmore M: Thoughts of harming infants in depressed and nondepressed mothers. J Affect Disord 54(1–2):21–28, 1999 10403143

Johnson A, Gesalman VE, Smith VE, et al: Motherhood and murder. Newsweek 138(1):20–25, 2001 11447810

Jones A: Women Who Kill. New York, The Feminist Press at the City University of New York, 1980

Kadushin A, Martin J: Child Abuse: An Interactional Event. New York, Columbus University Press, 1981

Kaplun D, Reich R: The murdered child and his killers. Am J Psychiatry 133(7):809–813, 1976 937572

Kempe CH, Silverman FN, Steele BF, et al: The battered-child syndrome. JAMA 181:17–24, 1962 14455086

Kendell RE, Chalmers JC, Platz C: Epidemiology of puerperal psychoses. Br J Psychiatry 150:662–673, 1987 3651704

Knops GG: Postpartum mood disorders. A startling contrast to the joy of birth. Postgrad Med 93(3):103–104, 109–110, 113–116, 1993 8446520

Kunz J, Bahr SJ: A profile of parental homicide against children. J Fam Violence 11(4):347–362, 1996

Levitzky S, Cooper R: Infant colic syndrome—maternal fantasies of aggression and infanticide. Clin Pediatr (Phila) 39(7):395–400, 2000 10914303

Lewis CF, Resnick PJ: Infanticide and neonaticide, in Violence in America: An Encyclopedia, Vol 2. Edited by Gottesman R, Brown RM. New York, Charles Scribner's Sons, 1999, pp 171–174

Mariano TY, Chan HC, Myers WC: Toward a more holistic understanding of filicide: a multidisciplinary analysis of 32 years of U.S. arrest data. Forensic Sci Int 236:46–53, 2014 24529774

Marks MN: Characteristics and causes of infanticide in Britain. Int Rev Psychiatry 8(1):99–106, 1996

Marleau JD, Poulin B, Webanck T, et al: Paternal filicide: a study of 10 men. Can J Psychiatry 44(1):57–63, 1999 10076742

McDermaid G, Winkler EG: Psychopathology of infanticide. J Clin Exp Psychopathol 16(1):22–41, 1955 14367503

Meyer CL, Oberman M, White K, et al: Mothers Who Kill Their Children: Understanding the Acts of Moms from Susan Smith to the "Prom Mom." New York, New York University Press, 2001

Morton JH: Female homicides. J Ment Sci 80:64–74, 1934

Mowbray CT, Oyserman D, Bybee D, et al: Life circumstances of mothers with serious mental illnesses. Psychiatr Rehabil J 25(2):114–123, 2001 11769977

Nonacs R, Cohen LS: Postpartum mood disorders: diagnosis and treatment guidelines. J Clin Psychiatry 59(suppl 2):34–40, 1998 9559758

Oates W, O'Neill E (eds): Medea by Euripides, in The Complete Greek Drama, Vol 1, New York, Random House, 1938

Oberman M: Mothers who kill: coming to terms with modern American infanticide. Am Crim Law Rev 34:1–110, 1996

Overpeck MD, Brenner RA, Trumble AC, et al: Risk factors for infant homicide in the United States. N Engl J Med 339(17):1211–1216, 1998 9780342

Pagelow MD: Family Violence. New York, Praeger, 1984

Perlin ML: The Jurisprudence of the Insanity Defense. Durham, NC, Carolina Academic Press, 1994

Resnick PJ: Child murder by parents: a psychiatric review of filicide. Am J Psychiatry 126(3):325–334, 1969 5801251

Resnick PJ: The Andrea Yates case: insanity on trial. Clevel State Law Rev 55(2):147–156, 2007

Ryan D, Milis L, Misri N: Depression during pregnancy. Can Fam Physician 51:1087–1093, 2005 16121830

Rynearson EK: Bereavement after homicide: a descriptive study. Am J Psychiatry 141(11):1452–1454, 1984 6496791

Shelton JL, Muirhead Y, Canning KE: Ambivalence toward mothers who kill: an examination of 45 U.S. cases of maternal neonaticide. Behav Sci Law 28(6):812–831, 2010 21110394

Sit D, Rothschild AJ, Wisner KL: A review of postpartum psychosis. J Womens Health (Larchmt) 15(4):352–368, 2006 16724884

Stanton J, Simpson A, Wouldes T: A qualitative study of filicide by mentally ill mothers. Child Abuse Negl 24(11):1451–1460, 2000 11128176

Smith D: Mom convicted of murder in 2011 killing of infant daughter. The Sacramento Bee, November 13, 2015

Stowe ZN, Calhoun K, Ramsey C, et al: Mood disorders during pregnancy and lactation: defining issues of exposure and treatment. CNS Spectr 6(2):150–166, 2001

Terp IM, Mortensen PB: Post-partum psychoses. Clinical diagnoses and relative risk of admission after parturition. Br J Psychiatry 172:521–526, 1998 9828994

Thomas C, Adshead G, Mezey G: Case report: traumatic responses to child murder. The Journal of Forensic Psychiatry 5(1):168–176, 1994

Tuteur W, Glotzer J: Murdering mothers. Am J Psychiatry 116:447–452, 1959 13840024

West SG, Friedman SH, Resnick PJ: Fathers who kill their children: an analysis of the literature. J Forensic Sci 54(2):463–468, 2009 19187457

Wilczynski A: Child Homicide. London, Oxford University Press, 1997

Wisner KL, Peindl KS, Gigliotti T, et al: Obsessions and compulsions in women with postpartum depression. J Clin Psychiatry 60(3):176–180, 1999 10192593

7

Siblicide

Jacqueline Landess, M.D., J.D.

INTRODUCTION: "THE DEVIL WAS IN ME"

On the morning of January 21, 2014, 14-year-old Alicia (a pseudonym, as she was a juvenile at the time of the crime) entered the bedroom of her 11-year-old half-sister, Dora, and stabbed her approximately 40 times with a kitchen knife. Dora died from wounds to her neck, chest, and arms (Mungin 2014). The crime shocked the small community of Mundelein, Illinois, a Chicago suburb where homicides rarely occur.

Superficially, Alicia and Dora appeared to be loving sisters who enjoyed each other's company. Neighbor Matthew McCoy reflected, "They would play in the front yard often. The oldest girl would help the young girl do cartwheels" (Black et al. 2014). Liam Welch, one of Alicia's former classmates, observed that Alicia was "funny and caring" and was "always there" for friends in need (Black et al. 2014). Alicia's attorney provided some insight as to what may have gone awry in the time preceding the tragic murder. Michael Conway reported that Alicia had taken on many adult responsibilities while her mother, a single parent, worked several jobs. She was reported to be in counseling at age 11 after waving a baseball bat at her mother (Black 2015).

Alicia reported that she stabbed Dora because she felt that her sister was ungrateful for all that she had done recently. Alicia had cooked dinner six times the week before and done a number of household chores. She also reported that Dora had recently hit her (Mungin 2014). Assistant State Attorney Claudia Kasten stated, "[Alicia] indicated that she was mad from the night before. She went downstairs and got a kitchen knife…with each stab wound she said [Dora] was not thankful for what she (the older sister) had done" (Huffpost 2014).

After the attack, Alicia took a shower and called 911, reporting that she had been awakened by her sister's screams and observed a Hispanic man fleeing the home (Bacon 2014). She later confessed to the crime when police informed her they had strands of hair in evidence that would lead them to the suspect (NBC Chicago 2015). In a two-page written statement to the police, Alicia said, "My mind was in another place and the devil was in me, and that is why my sister…is dead" (Black 2015).

Alicia pled guilty to first-degree murder (Black 2015). Her case was adjudicated in juvenile court, and she was offered a plea bargain in which she will remain in a juvenile detention facility until she turns 21, with the possibility of parole within 5 years of her sentencing (Black 2015). Alicia expressed remorse at her sentencing. She stated, "I am truly sorry for the pain I have caused [my mother and stepfather]." She reflected on how she and Dora used to make bracelets together, play sports, and watch movies: "I can never get [those times] back." She stated her future plans included finishing high school and pursuing a career in nursing. Mr. Conway, her attorney, expressed faith that the teen could be rehabilitated, stating, "What happened a little over a year ago…is not who she is. It was an aberration" (Black 2015).

OVERVIEW

Siblicide (also referred to as *fratricide*) is defined as the killing of one's sibling. Historically, famous examples abound in which siblings kill each other out of rage, resentment, jealousy, and impulsivity. Biblically, the first murder occurred with Cain killing his younger brother Abel out of envy and rage. Claudius poisoned King Hamlet, his brother, and married Hamlet's widow to obtain the throne of Denmark. Genghis Khan allegedly murdered his older half-brother during a conflict over food. In Greek mythology, Medea killed her brother, Apsyrtus, as she and Jason fled with the golden fleece, dismembering him and scattering the parts so her father would be distracted in gathering his limbs and delayed in pursuing her.

Although violence between siblings is the most common form of intrafamilial violence, siblicide itself is a rare phenomenon, estimated to represent less than 2% of homicides (Bourget and Gagné 2006; Ewing 1997). When it does occur, the tragedy often is sensationalized and becomes national news, particularly when the case involves juvenile siblings. Adult siblicides, however, account for the majority of cases (Gebo 2002; Marleau and Saucier 1998; Underwood and Patch 1999).

In part because of its rarity, there is a dearth of literature and research devoted to sibling murders. The research that exists is limited by small sample sizes and inadequate databases, which commonly lead to limited generalizability in conclusions. Most studies are descriptive in nature. Various theories exist regarding seniority, motivations, and contributing factors, but no one theory has been necessarily "proven" or debunked given the limited statistical power of most studies.

Although juvenile siblicides cannot be categorically differentiated from adult siblicides, some studies have found differences in seniority (whether younger or older sibling is the perpetrator) and motive (Daly et al. 2001). Juvenile perpetrators often kill impulsively in the context of seemingly minor disagreements, perhaps in the setting of long-standing rivalry. Juvenile siblicides also occur in the context of negligence, such as accidental discharge of a firearm or fire setting. Adult siblicides tend to revolve around issues of money, property, and power. Few studies have been able to convincingly analyze differences in motive and prevalence of siblicide in regard to genetic relatedness (half-sibling vs. full sibling relationship).

In sum, the topic of siblicide is understudied and thus poorly understood. With few exceptions, the existing literature must be approached as an attempt to understand what is presently known about the epidemiology, motives, and dynamics of sibling murders but cannot be generalized to all, or even most, siblicides.

EPIDEMIOLOGY

Sibling Aggression

Using Uniform Crime Reporting data, Underwood and Patch (1999) determined that siblicides account for 1 of every 100 homicides, making it a rare form of family homicide. In contrast, rates of nonhomicide sibling violence are higher than those for any other form of intrafamilial violence (Hoffman et al. 2005). Classically written off as "sibling rivalry," aggression between siblings, particularly during childhood, is viewed as a normative, necessary phase of development and maturity, with parents often viewing sibling conflict as a "learning ground" for later social interactions (Krienert and Walsh 2011). Factors such as temperament, gender, relatedness, birth order/spacing, and perceived parental favoritism all contribute to the likelihood of aggression between siblings (Salmon and Hehman 2014). From toddlerhood onward, fights over personal space and possessions cause the most frequent and intense conflicts (McGuire et al. 2000).

Parents, society, and the justice system tend to decriminalize or minimize altercations that would amount to assault or worse if perpetrated by unrelated individuals. While benefits of sibling conflict include greater capacity to empathize and problem solve in difficult social situations, unmitigated sibling conflict can result in a host of behavioral and psychological problems if left unchecked (Salmon and Hehman 2014). Even siblings themselves may minimize the quality and effects of sibling violence. In a retrospective study of 203 undergraduate students, 50% reported a history of sibling physical aggression, but only 10% viewed the aggression as abusive (Hardy 2001). While most aggression is commonly perpetrated by pushing/shoving with hands or feet and results in minor injury, instances of more serious injury do occur (Krienert and Walsh 2011). Krienert and Walsh (2011) analyzed U.S. Federal Bureau of Investigation data involving 33,066 cases of sibling assaults in which the victim and offender were 21 years or younger and determined that 3.1% of sibling assaults resulted in major injury. This study also found that male abusers with female victims were most common. When it came to more serious assaults, females were more likely to use knives, whereas males preferred firearms (Krienert and Walsh 2011). Aggression has also been found to be most frequent when the age difference between offender and victim is less than 3 years, suggesting jealousy and time together as contributing factors (Felson and Russo 1988). Physical aggression toward siblings does decrease with age, but it does not entirely resolve with increased maturity, as nearly two-thirds of teens ages 15–17 have hit a brother or sister at least once in the past year (Straus et al. 2006). Ultimately, however, it is unknown if sibling violence predisposes to siblicide, given that sibling aggression is so common, whereas siblicide itself is rare.

Age and Seniority

Although juvenile murders receive more media coverage, adult siblicides account for more than 75% of cases (Ewing 1997; Gebo 2002; Marleau and Saucier 1998). Most siblicides occur in early to middle adulthood

(Dawson and Langan 1994); one study found the average age of offender and victim to be 34 and 33, respectively (Underwood and Patch 1999). Sibling murders have been found to occur most often when the victim and offender are fewer than 5 years apart; this finding bolsters the validity of theories that posit these violent conflicts are provoked in part by competition for limited parental attention and resources (Daly et al. 2001; Marleau 2005). Another factor contributing to conflict may be related to siblings fewer than 5 years apart spending more time together than siblings separated by larger age gaps.

In nonhumans, birth order and siblicidal behaviors are related. Particularly among avian species, siblicidal behavior is not uncommon. Some birds, such as the black eagle, engage in obligate siblicide, meaning that the bigger, stronger chick (usually the eldest) will kill the youngest despite availability of food resources. However, other species (e.g., ospreys, hyenas) engage in facultative siblicide, in which the killing of a sibling is dependent on availability of scarce nutritional resources (Salmon and Hehman 2014). Sulloway (1996) has posited that evolutionary theories extend to human siblicides as well. Using a Darwinian approach, he predicted younger siblings were less likely to kill elder siblings because doing so would compromise the younger sibling's inclusive fitness. He hypothesized that because elder siblings generally reproduce before younger siblings, a younger sibling would jeopardize the survival of existing nieces and nephews if the younger sibling killed the elder one (Sulloway 1996). Several studies have found elder human siblings kill younger siblings more often in childhood but that the reverse holds true in adulthood (Daly et al. 2001; Gebo 2002). Notwithstanding evolutionary hypotheses, several factors may explain this finding. First, the likelihood of killing anyone increases when aging from adolescence to adulthood. The other obvious factor may be that in childhood, older siblings are likely to be bigger and stronger and to have more access to certain weapons compared with younger siblings. In adult siblicides, younger brothers or sisters are more likely to murder older siblings (Daly et al. 2001; Marleau 2005). Younger siblings may be more likely to kill their older siblings in adulthood because of resentment of authority or longtime power struggles, usually exacerbated by acute conflict (Ewing 1997).

Gender and Race

Males are most likely to be both offenders and victims (Gebo 2002; Underwood and Patch 1999). More specifically, in the case of juvenile siblicides, males have been found to be four times more likely than females to kill a sibling (Peck and Heide 2012). However, "female-on-female homicides are 40% more likely to occur in the sibling relationship than in any non-familial relationship" (Gebo 2002, p. 162). In decreasing order, the most common combinations of siblicides are the following: brother offender and victim, brother offender and sister victim, sister offender and brother victim, and sister offender and victim (Gebo 2002; Peck and Heide 2012). In the United States, the majority of siblicides occur among whites and blacks, but Native Americans have the highest rates of siblicide than any other racial/ethnic group (Gebo 2002). This could be due to the increased number of siblings in many Native American households, higher rates of poverty, and higher rates of substance abuse (see discussion of associations with substance use later in this chapter) in this population.

Use of Weapon

Underwood and Patch (1999) found that the most prevalent weapon used in U.S. siblicides was a firearm (59%), followed by knives or other cutting instruments. In contrast, Bourget and Gagné (2006) found that most Canadian siblicide deaths had been due to stabbing (70%), followed by shooting and beating. This difference in weapon choice is likely related to the increased availability of firearms in the United States compared with Canada. Overall, males were more likely to use firearms in acts of abuse or violence, compared with female counterparts.

Presence of Mental Illness and Substance Use

The association of mental illness with siblicide is unclear because of limited data. Using coroners' files, Bourget and Gagné (2006) conducted an analysis of 10 (mostly adult) siblicides that occurred in Canada over 9 years and found that one-third of the offenders were mentally ill at the time of the offense and that most had no history of a prior criminal record. In this study, alcohol was found to play a role in 60% of offenses. Others have found alcohol to play a critical role as well, particularly in adult siblicides (Ewing 1997). In one case, an adult man turned on his brother after a 2-day binge on alcohol, diazepam, and cocaine. The judge noted that in his experience, "these cases tend to arise from an alcohol-fueled" fight between family members (The Irish Times 2008).

Bender's analysis of juvenile homicide offenders (some who committed fratricide) found that nearly all had psychiatric or neuropsychiatric issues, such as brain damage, intellectual disability, epilepsy, or schizophrenia (Bender 1959). However, others have noted that among children who murder, particularly those of preadolescent age, their behavior usually reflects "immaturity, rage, and poor impulse control" rather than a serious psychiatric disturbance (Adam and Livingston 1993, p. 50). For example, a 10-year-old girl who killed her 7-year-old sister had narcissistic, antisocial, and obsessive traits and likely had had anger and resentment toward her younger sister for years (Adam and Livingston 1993).

Summary

Although extensive data are lacking, the most common characteristics of a siblicide are that the victim and offender are male and of adult age, the younger sibling kills the older, and, in the United States, the offender most likely uses a firearm. Psychosis and substance use are risk factors. Personality traits, external stressors, birth order, and temperament play a role in sibling violence as well.

TYPES OF HOMICIDES

Accidental Deaths

Minor siblings who kill their brothers or sisters often do so accidentally, although no aggregate data exist comparing accidental and intentional siblicides. Many accidental deaths are due to lack of firearm safety. A fairly typical example occurred recently in Chicago, Illinois. Israel LaSalle was in another room of the home while his grandsons played "cops and robbers." His 6-year-old grandson grabbed a gun from the top of a refrigerator and the gun went off, striking and killing his 3-year-old brother. Mr. LaSalle was unaware of the gun's presence in the home, and the boys' father ultimately faced felony child endangerment charges. The father had recently showed the gun to his 6-year-old and instructed him that it was only for adult use (Flores et al. 2015).

Some studies have asserted that existing Centers for Disease Control and Prevention data on the accidental shooting of children by firearms underestimate the true number of deaths (Foley 2016; Hemenway and Solnick 2015; Luo and McIntire 2013). This presumed underestimation is due to inconsistent classification of deaths as homicides by coroners. For instance, a shooter may intentionally pull the trigger, believing the gun is not loaded, or simply not understand how the gun works. Despite the shooter's lack of intent, the shooting may still be classified as a homicide, meaning death at the hands of another. Of course, in some cases it is unknown whether the child had intent to kill, and while some children have been charged with manslaughter or worse, often the parent or guardian bears responsibility for the death of the child in their care.

One study examined data from 16 states over an 8-year period in which a child was either a victim or a shooter. In the age group from birth to 14 years old, 229 unintentional firearm deaths were identified. Approximately two-thirds of these deaths were other-inflicted; of these, approximately 61% of shooters were family members and 30% were friends. Of family member–involved shootings, brothers were most commonly the shooter (Hemenway and Solnick 2015). One-half of shooting accidents occur at home, and another one-third occur at a friend's house (Luo and McIntire 2013). Primary factors related to accidental shootings appear to be lack of parental supervision or neglect, ready access to firearms, curiosity, and peer influences. At times, substance use and/or emotional issues play a role as well.

Of course, there are other methods in which a sibling accidentally kills a brother or sister. Children's fascination with fire and fire-setting may lead to calamitous results. Jacob Morgan was 17 years old when he was accused of murder and arson in the death of his 14-month-old half-brother. Jacob had a history of learning disabilities and mental health problems and allegedly had a fascination with fire. According to news reports, Jacob lit tea candles throughout the home while babysitting his baby brother. He was then unable to put out the resulting blaze. Although it was acknowledged that Jacob may have had no intent to kill his brother, he was sentenced to 15 years in prison (Southmayd 2015; WBTV Web Staff 2016).

Intentional Homicides

In adults, siblicides result from perhaps longer-standing tensions that erupt into acute conflict often in the context of substance use and usually over property, money, and/or responsibilities; however, these characteristics share commonalities with homicide generally (Bourget and Gagné 2006; Ewing 1997). Multiple reports describe siblings who are forced to live together because of stressors and vulnerabilities such as financial deprivation, poverty, divorce, mental health issues, and illness. Oftentimes, these siblings experience mounting tensions, and one turns on the other in the context of minor conflicts.

In juveniles, motivations often appear to stem from perceived parental favoritism, envy, jealousy, and competition for limited resources (attention, sharing of responsibilities), as well as emotional and behavioral disturbances. As Charles Ewing, a forensic psychologist at the University of Buffalo, observes, "Siblings can have very conflicted relationships, and of all the familial relationships, siblings are the most competitive—for status, for power, for affection, for space within the home and family" (quoted in Booth 1998). Oftentimes, firstborns are particularly sensitive to feelings of displacement and competition when a younger sibling comes into the picture.

A 10-year-old girl who killed her 7-year-old sister demonstrated these elements of jealousy and resentment (Adam and Livingston 1993). The family had moved 3 years earlier, and the older girl was having difficulty adjusting. She had fewer friends than her younger sister and was often expected to help her sister with homework. The older sister felt her younger sister was her father's "favorite." The younger sibling had hit her and called her names in the past, most recently the day before the murder. Marital conflict also allegedly played a role in general household tension. The older child ultimately stabbed her younger sister to death during a 10-minute unsupervised period while their father was returning from work (Adam and Livingston 1993).

Parents may negligently fail to intervene before violence escalates. Walsh and Krienert (2014) hypothesized that elements of chronic and acute strain may contribute to siblicides, and the differential gender response to stress (males tending to externalize more than females) may explain why male siblicide offenders predominate. Analyzing national data of siblicide victim and offenders age 21 or younger, they found that males most often killed in the context of an argument, which is typical of adolescent male violence generally.

Although working from a small sample size composed of individuals ages 17–55, Bourget and Gagné (2006) identified two subtypes of siblicides. The first subtype comprised impulsive, unplanned acts of violence, stemming from a disagreement often in context of alcohol abuse. These murders accounted for 60% of fratricides. The authors hypothesized that these murders "might ultimately represent an extreme manifestation of sibling dynamics with high expressed emotions and some degree of rivalry" (p. 533). The second subtype involved "disordered psychotic behavior" and premeditated homicide. As Bourget and Gagné observed, "Psychotic fratricides were associated with a drive to exterminate the family, extending beyond the killing of the sibling to incorporate the killing of at least one parent" (p. 533).

UNIQUE ASSESSMENT ISSUES

A thorough evaluation of a siblicide offender should include not only a description of psychiatric illness but also identification of chronic emotional states and stressors that may have led to the homicide. Especially in adult siblicides, a careful substance history should be obtained to determine the effects that alcohol or drug intoxication may have had in accelerating a conflict.

Ascertaining whether the offender has a history of violence, as well as a history of escalating violence toward the victim, is critical. While it is not entirely clear how to interpret acts of nonlethal violence toward a sibling that occur during childhood, it would seem logical to infer that repeated, predatory, and nonreactive threats and assaults against a sibling could be seen as bullying at best and a precursor for more lethal violence at worst. In addition, children who demonstrate high levels of impulsive aggression and disinhibition should be assessed and treated. While untreated impulsivity alone may not result in lethal violence, an impulsive, disinhibited sibling who has accessibility to lethal weapons, lack of parental supervision, and conflict with a sibling may be more predisposed to reactively assault or injure a sibling.

In children, the determination of whether a death was accidental or purposeful can be challenging. Purposeful acts may occur but without malice; for instance, a preadolescent boy may intentionally pull a gun's trigger while pointing the weapon at his sibling but may have believed the gun was not loaded. Oftentimes, in these cases parents or caregivers are prosecuted following the death (see section "Prevention" later in this chapter). The infancy defense descended from British common law and held that children under the age of 7 were incapable of forming criminal intent. Statutes vary across jurisdictions, but generally, in criminal cases, children under the age of 7 (and in some states, under the age of 10) are barred from prosecution. Many juvenile courts, however, reject the infancy defense, deeming it unnecessary given the protective, rehabilitative goals of the juvenile court (Bazelon 2000). There has been a shift away from harsh punishment of juveniles who commit homicides and other serious crimes. The Supreme Court held that mandatory life sentences without parole and the death penalty for juveniles are both unconstitutional, recognizing the impact of immature brain development, impulsivity, peer influence, and thrill seeking on children's behaviors (*Miller v. Alabama* 2012; *Roper v. Simmons* 2005).

AFTERMATH

The effects of siblicide are particularly traumatic for parents and the remaining brothers and sisters. Parents, already facing the loss of one child, often have no choice about whether the accused child is prosecuted, even if the killing may have been accidental. Parents are in an agonizing and unenviable position: one child is dead, and the other is sent to prison. In addition, the accused may experience posttraumatic symptoms, guilt, and remorse. If left unaddressed, this could lead to a lifetime of psychological problems.

PREVENTION

Juvenile Siblicides

Risk factors in juvenile siblicides commonly involve a lack of parental supervision, siblings who are close in age competing for limited resources (time, property, personal space, responsibilities, friends), available weapons, and opportunity. Murders occurring during fits of rage, set off by seemingly minor disagreements, are not uncommon. Although it seems logical to conclude that siblicide is an extreme manifestation of sibling rivalry, it is simply too rare of a phenomenon to conclusively make this statement. However, because past violence is a predictor of future violence, it seems logical that escalating sibling aggression should certainly be seen as a potential warning sign of more serious violent acts.

Prevention efforts should focus on proactively addressing sibling violence and educating families about the harmful effects of physical and emotional aggression between siblings. Conflict resolution skills should be taught and modeled. Particular attention should be paid to siblings who, because of temperament or personality, may be less resilient and more vulnerable to stress. Many family systems in which juvenile siblicides occur are also under strain, whether it be from poverty, marital woes, mental illness, or other conflict within the home. Strengthening these systems as a whole, by improving parents' emotional capacity and availability to their children, would likely decrease acts of violence generally.

The most common weapon used in siblicides (at least among U.S. males) is a firearm. Some states have enacted laws that impose criminal liability upon gun owners when minors access guns. Twenty-seven states have child access prevention laws, which impose criminal liability on gun owners if a child accesses their firearms (Washington State Legislature 2017). However, access is not strictly defined, and exceptions apply. Some states penalize gun owners who directly provide guns to minors, while the strictest statutes impose liability when a minor gains access to negligently stored firearms. In regard to gun storage, 11 states have laws concerning firearm-locking devices; Massachusetts is the only state to require that guns be stored with a locking device in place. Of course, in cases of accidental shootings, parents or caregivers can be charged with a range of crimes: child endangerment with or without serious injury, involuntary manslaughter, and child neglect. These crimes range from misdemeanors and felonies with commensurate penalties extending from probation and fines to lengthy prison sentences.

Although gun laws and gun safety are at times contentious, politicized topics, a host of shooting deaths committed by children could likely have been prevented by decreased access to firearms. Parents should be informed of the data and risks to their children if firearms are left unattended.

Adult Siblicides

Substances, particularly alcohol, are involved in a number of adult siblicides. Scenarios often involve adult siblings in close proximity (spending increased time together or living under the same roof) who engage in a heated argument and violence ensues. Long-standing tensions, rivalries, and conflicts may come to a head. In at least some cases, untreated mental illness plays a role. In Bourget and Gagné's (2006) sample, three cases involved premeditated homicide with psychotic intent.

Given these scenarios, prevention should address alcoholism and substance use disorders within family systems. A treating clinician should also pay close attention to chronic stress, jealousy, envy, and rivalries between siblings. In the face of chronic conflict, an acute precipitant, even if minor, may trigger a sequence of events that end in homicide. The vulnerabilities of the individual sibling to rejection, favoritism, stress, and neglect should be identified. Preventive efforts should focus on teaching prosocial responses to conflict and stress, addressing substance use, and improving self-esteem of the individual sibling.

CONCLUSION

Sibling rivalry is nearly universal, and children and adolescents are far more impulsive and less inhibited than adults, in part because of immature brain development. Despite these factors, siblicide is a rare occurrence. Small sample sizes lead to limited generalizability of results. However, certain epidemiological trends have been observed in multiple studies: adult siblings tend to kill each other more often than juvenile siblings, and brothers kill brothers with the highest frequency. Motivations in sibling homicides vary, but chronic states of envy, jealousy, resentment, and competition, when fueled by substances and acute stressors or conflict, may culminate in murderous acts. In terms of prevention, juvenile siblicides could likely be decreased through a combination of increased parental supervision, decreased access to weapons, and early interventions in escalating sibling violence. Efforts to reduce adult siblicides must include treatment of substance use, mental illness, chronic stress, and simmering family conflicts.

REFERENCES

Adam BS, Livingston R: Sororicide in preteen girls. A case report and literature review. Acta Paedopsychiatr 56(1):47–51, 1993 8517161

Bacon J: Illinois teen accused in stabbing death of sister, 11. USA Today, January 23, 2014

Bazelon, LA: Exploding the superpredator myth: why infancy is the preadolescent's best defense in juvenile court. NYU Law Review 75(159):190–198, 2000

Bender L: Children and adolescents who have killed. Am J Psychiatry 116:510–513, 1959

Black L: Mundelein teen sentenced in stabbing death of sister. Chicago Tribune, March 3, 2015

Black L, Keilman J, Waters D: Police say sibling dispute turned deadly: "She kept stabbing." Chicago Tribune, January 23, 2014

Booth W: Girls' murder focuses light on hidden specter of sibling abuse. The Washington Post, August 14, 1998

Bourget D, Gagné P: Fratricide: a forensic psychiatric perspective. J Am Acad Psychiatry Law 34(4):529–533, 2006 17185484

Daly M, Wilson M, Salmon CA, et al: Siblicide and seniority. Homicide Stud 5(1):30–45, 2001

Dawson JM, Langan PA: Murder in Families. Washington, DC, Bureau of Justice Statistics, 1994

Ewing CP: Fatal Families: The Dynamics of Intrafamilial Homicide. Thousand Oaks, CA, Sage, 1997, pp 115–126

Felson RB, Russo NF: Parental punishment and sibling aggression. Soc Psychol Q 51(1):11–18, 1988

Flores R, Pearson M, Sutton J: Charges against Chicago dad after 6-year-old shoots 3-year-old. CNN, October 19, 2015

Foley R: New CDC data understate accidental shooting deaths of kids. USA Today, December 9, 2016

Gebo E: A contextual exploration of siblicide. Violence Vict 17(2):157–168, 2002 12033552

Hardy MS: Physical aggression and sexual behavior among siblings: a retrospective study. J Fam Violence 16(3):255–268, 2001

Hemenway D, Solnick SJ: Children and unintentional firearm death. Inj Epidemiol 2(1):26, 2015 26478854

Hoffman KL, Kiecolt J, Edwards JN: Physical violence between siblings: a theoretical and empirical analysis. J Fam Issues 26(8):1103–1130, 2005

Huffpost: 14-year-old Mundelein girl charged with murder of 11-year-old half-sister. Huffingtonpost.com, January 23, 2014. Available at: http://www.huffingtonpost.com/2014/01/22/mundelein-murder_n_4645251.html. Accessed January 6, 2017.

The Irish Times: Dublin man jailed for 4 1/2 years for killing brother. The Irish Times (website), October 14, 2008. Available at: http://www.irishtimes.com/news/dublin-man-jailed-for-4-1-2-years-for-killing-brother-1.830145. Accessed April 25, 2017.

Krienert J, Walsh J: My brother's keeper: a contemporary examination of reported sibling violence using national level data, 2000–2005. Journal of Family Violence 26(5):331–342, 2011

Luo M, McIntire M: Children and guns: the hidden toll. The New York Times, September 28, 2013

Marleau JD: Birth order and fratricide: an evaluation of Sulloway's hypothesis. Med Sci Law 45(1):52–56, 2005 15745274

Marleau JD, Saucier JF: Birth order and fratricidal behaviour in Canada. Psychol Rep 82(3 Pt 1):817–818, 1998 9676492

McGuire S, Manke B, Eftekhari A, et al: Children's perceptions of sibling conflict during middle childhood: issues and sibling (dis)similarity. Soc Dev 9(2):173–190, 2000

Miller v Alabama, 567 U.S. 460 (2012)

Mungin L: Police: girl, 14, stabs sister 40 times because she felt unappreciated. CNN, January 23, 2014

NBC Chicago: Mundelein girl charged in sister's stabbing offered a plea deal. NBC Chicago website, January 19, 2015. Available at: http://www.nbcchicago.com/news/local/Mundelein-Girl-Charged-in-Sisters-Stabbing-Offered-Plea-Deal-289075181.html. Accessed January 4, 2017.

Peck J, Heide K: Juvenile involvement in fratricide and sororicide: an empirical analysis of 32 years of U.S. arrest data. Journal of Family Violence 27(8):749–760, 2012

Roper v Simmons, 543 U.S. 551 (2005)

Salmon C, Hehman J: The evolutionary psychology of sibling conflict and siblicide, in The Evolution of Violence. New York, Springer, 2014, pp 137–157

Southmayd R: Family defends teen accused of killing 14-month-old half-brother near Lesslie. The Herald, March 11, 2015. Available at: http://www.heraldonline.com/news/local/crime/article13635782.html. Accessed April 25, 2017.

Straus MA, Gelles RJ, Steinmetz SK: Behind Closed Doors: Violence in the American Family. New York, Doubleday, 2006

Sulloway F: Birth order and personality, in Born to Rebel: Birth Order, Family Dynamics and Creative Lives. New York, Vintage Books, 1996, pp 55–82

Underwood R, Patch P: Siblicide: a descriptive analysis of sibling homicide. Homicide Stud 3(4):333–348, 1999

Walsh J, Krienert, J: My brother's reaper: examining officially reported siblicide incidents in the United States, 2000–2007. Violence Vict 29(3):523–540, 2014 25069154

Washington State Legislature: Summary of State Child Access Prevention Laws, 2017. Available at: http://leg.wa.gov/Senate/Committees/LAW/Documents/SummaryOfStateChildAccessPreventionLaws.pdf. Accessed April 25, 2017.

WBTV Web Staff: SC teen gets 15 years in baby half brother's death. February 10, 2016. Available at: http://wncn.com/2016/02/10/sc-teen-gets-15-years-in-baby-half-brothers-death/. Accessed April 25, 2017.

8

Parricide

Debra A. Pinals, M.D.

INTRODUCTION

Case 1: Lyle and Erik Menendez

On a summer evening in 1989, in a wealthy neighborhood of Beverly Hills, California, Joseph "Lyle" Menendez, age 21, and his brother Erik, age 18, shot their father and their mother, including a shot to the back of their father's head and gunshots to their kneecaps (Davis 1994). After the killings, the sons disposed of the guns they used and spent months traveling and spending large sums of money, living lavish lifestyles. They had been fortunate to have been among the wealthy elite, yet the crime was a mystery. The murders would eventually capture the imagination of the country—and of psychiatrists—as issues about their upbringing and their claimed motivations became a source of controversy and a strategy for their defense at trial. Evidence in question included statements confessing to the murders that Erik had made during the course of psychotherapy. The admissibility of those statements became fertile grounds for a legal struggle involving questions of confidentiality and privileged information at the criminal trial.

The legal debate about whether the psychologist's invocation of privilege on behalf of the Menendez brothers (that would have resulted in some information not being permitted at trial) would continue for over a year. Partially related to the issues raised from a threat made to the psychotherapist by Lyle, the Supreme Court of California ultimately allowed

113

some critical information from the therapy session to be introduced (*Menendez v. Superior Court* 1992). The trial was aired on television in 1993, during which evidence was introduced that the motive for the crime related to the sons' description of years of sexual and emotional abuse at the hands of their parents. This mitigating evidence was not persuasive to the jury, and they were each convicted and sentenced to life in prison. They remain incarcerated in the California prison system.

Case 2: The Parker-Hulme Murder

The Parker-Hulme murder of Honorah Parker in 1954 has left a haunting legacy in New Zealand (Gillies 2011). The murder is depicted in the 1994 popular film by Peter Jackson, *Heavenly Creatures*. In the actual case, two young women, Pauline Parker, age 16, and her friend Juliet Hulme, age 15, together conspired in the brutal killing of Pauline's mother. They bashed her head with a brick in a sock after walking with her on an outing to a secluded area. The court hearing and the public attention to the crime revealed allegations that the girls had engaged in some type of obsessive and possibly lesbian relationship. Psychiatrists testified that the girls had developed a shared paranoid belief system and were narcissistic and that their intensive attachment made them lose touch with reality. Juliet Hulme was scheduled to leave the country amid her parents' divorce and the parents growing concerns about the inseparable relationship between the girls. Although the girls wanted Pauline to join Juliet, the two girls believed Pauline's mother would not allow the trip. So, the girls took matters into their own hands. In her diary, Pauline described the plan they came up with to kill her mother amid descriptions of fun the two girls were having with each other (Parker 2014). The diary entries were used at trial. Pauline described the plan with odd enthusiasm and determination.

Pauline and Juliet unsuccessfully pled insanity. Their crime was ever more shocking as reports revealed the degree to which the girls seemed to take pride in the killing and totally lack remorse for the killing. This suggested, in retrospect, that the girls had become enveloped in an adolescent narcissistic fantasy world (Gillies 2011). Both girls were convicted of murder and spent 5 years incarcerated in separate facilities. Upon release, they were both allowed to leave New Zealand and established identities under different names. Juliet Hulme ultimately moved to Scotland, where she lives as Anne Perry and has become a best-selling crime novelist. Pauline Parker changed her name to Hilary Nathan and moved to England, where she lives a quiet, religious life in solitude.

OVERVIEW

The idea of killing a parent is nothing short of shocking. The traditional view of a parent reaping the rewards of raising children and watching them become contributing members of society is rocked by the thought of this gruesome ending of that parental dream. This chapter reviews this darker outcome for a parent that involves the rare and complicated phenomenon of a child (as a minor or as an adult) killing a parent.

Mythology is replete with stories of sons and daughters killing their parents. Emotions that include themes of sex, greed, anger, revenge, or control course through the stories of such incidents. Newhill (1991) provided a detailed overview of the topic of parricide and reviewed tales within mythology and the literature that encompass such incidents. For example, in Greek mythology, Oedipus kills his father and marries his mother, a story that has left its mark on countless writings related to incest and taboos of such relationships. Freud wrote of the Oedipus complex, the psychodynamic desire to kill the father to win the mother as an object of love and sexual partner. The Orestes complex derives from the tale of Orestes, who is persuaded by his sister Electra to kill their mother out of revenge for their mother's killing of their father. The Orestes complex relates to attachment to the mother and the lines between attachment and aggression. Freud's views intertwine sexual desire of one parent and the disdain for the other who stands in the way of achieving this desired pairing. Hillbrand et al. (1999) described the crime of parricide as having such a strong negative moral valence because it violates two basic societal rules: the rule of honoring one's parents and the prohibition against murder. These social edicts are sacred not only in Judeo-Christian teachings, so when they are broken, the response across society is extreme.

The general term that is used to describe killing one or both parents is *parricide. Matricide* is the killing of one's mother, and *patricide* is the specific term for the killing of one's father. Homicides of stepparents are also sometimes called *stepparricide*, although this distinction is not uniformly clear in the literature. Studies examining parricide at times exclude stepparricide, given the complex differences across those relationships, such as whether the stepparent raised the child or came into an individual's life much later. Thus, differences in dynamics usually make the phenomenon of stepparricide distinct from parricide. *Double parricide* describes the killing of both parents. Sometimes these crimes are associated with suicide or suicide attempts. Parricide that includes killing other family members may have different motives and often different dynamics; it is more commonly referred to as *familial homicide* or *family annihilation* (see Chapter 10 for further discussion). Parricide alone, like other intrafamilial murder, presents a window into complicated family dynamics and is generally the culmination of factors that may or may not have been recognized before the murder.

EPIDEMIOLOGY

In a review of clinical literature on the topic, Newhill (1991) described perpetrators of parricides across four broad categories of age, gender, victim, motivation, circumstances, and psychopathology. She looked at the following perpetrator victim combinations: 1) children/adolescents who kill their fathers; 2) children/adolescents who kill their mothers; 3) adult males who kill their parents, and especially those who kill their fathers; and 4) adult females who kill parents, and especially those who kill their mothers. These categorizations can be helpful in looking at some of the data on the frequency and characteristics of parricide.

Hillbrand et al. (1999) consolidated data and found that parricide accounts for about 2% of all homicides, with patricides outnumbering matricides and male perpetrators far outnumbering female perpetrators. This reflects a review of U.S. national crime data and consolidates several studies. Millaud et al. (1996) reported that parricides reflect 6.3% of homicides in Canada. Stoessel and Bornstein (1988) reported that parricides composed 2%–3% of homicides in France. Table 8–1 summarizes the rates of homicide (per 100,000 people) in 2000 across these studies. Two studies have cited data suggesting a downward trend in parricides across the United States (Shon and Targonski 2003; Walsh et al. 2008). Heide (1993a) reported that among intrafamilial murders, approximately 10% involve parricide. In a review of a national sample of cases examining homicide reports involving parricide offenders under age 21 between 1976 and 2003, Walsh et al. (2008) found that rates for white male offenders peak in late adolescence and those for white females peak in mid-adolescence. Biological fathers were at greatest risk of victimization, but girls were more likely than boys to kill a stepfather.

Another review of similar U.S. data examining offenders of all ages found that parents murdered by their children were on average in their mid-50s; the ages of victims ranged from late 20s to late 90s (Heide and Petee 2007). Males were significantly more likely than females to be perpetrators of both patricide and matricide (87% and 84%, respectively). Males also were more likely than females to commit double parricide. Offenders of patricide ranged in age from 7 to 72, and offenders of matricide ranged in age from 8 to 78 years old. The mean age of perpetrators of pat-

TABLE 8-1. Estimated parricide rates in the United States, Canada, and France based on homicide rates in 2000

	Homicide rate per 100,000[a]	Parricide rate (% parricide among homicides)
United States	5.8%	0.116% (2.0%)
Canada	1.8%	0.1056% (5.9%)
France	1.8%	0.045% (2.5%)

[a]Homicide rate per 100,000 estimated from United Nations Development Reports, available at http://hdr.undp.org/en/content/homicide-rate-100000.
Source. Data from Hillbrand et al. 1999; Millaud et al. 1996; Stoessel and Bornstein 1988.

ricide was slightly younger, at 25 years, than perpetrators of matricide, at 30 years. Interestingly, however, nearly three-quarters (72%) of the patricides involved perpetrators under 30 years old, and 91% involved perpetrators under 40 years of age. For matricide, the offenders skewed toward being older, with 56% of offenders being under 30 years old and 91% being under 50 years of age. Juvenile perpetrators represented a substantial minority of offenders, with one in four patricides and one in six matricides being perpetrated by individuals younger than 18 years.

Heide and Petee (2007) provided a further delineation of the circumstances surrounding the killing of parents. Although the U.S. Federal Bureau of Investigation Supplemental Homicide Report database used in this research has limitations in its classifications of circumstances, it appears that 86% of mothers and fathers were killed in incidents involving single victims and single offenders. The remaining 14% were killed in multiple-victim circumstances (a small percentage of which involved nonparents). There were six main categories delineating the circumstances of murder in this database, and for parricide a narrow majority (52%) involved situations involving "other argument." This was more likely for fathers as victims (58%) than for mothers as victims (44%). Mothers were more likely to be killed in circumstances described as "other nonfelony"—related reasons or in circumstances that could not be determined. The authors concluded that overall, arguments are common precursors to parricide, especially arguments related to money and property or involving alcohol.

Other analysis of U.S. data by Heide (1993b) sheds some light on the methods used in parricide. The use of a firearm was the most common means of killing a father in this analysis. Other means more likely used to kill mothers included cutting, blunt instruments, or straight assaults, whereas firearms were more commonly used by juveniles than by adults in parent killings. Green (1981) found that asphyxiation was another common means of killing mothers. Green also found that in 95% of cases reviewed, the parricide took place in the home.

International comparisons can be helpful, especially because firearms access is different across countries. Canadian coroner file data from 1990 to 2005 revealed 64 cases of parricide out of 720 domestic homicides (9%; Bourget et al. 2007). Here again, sons were more likely to be perpetrators than daughters. Sons were more likely to use blunt instruments in matricide, followed by knives, whereas for patricide, knives, followed by firearms, were most likely to be used. Homicide-suicides were seen in almost a third of the matricide cases and almost 17% of the patricide cases among the sons who perpetrated the parricide (because of the low base rate of daughter-perpetrated parricide, data were only available for sons). In eight of the parricides, the parents' bodies were decapitated or mutilated, including genital mutilation. In five of the eight such instances, of the people who engaged in mutilation, the perpetrator was psychotic. *Overkill*—the use of an excessive amount of violence in the murder—was seen in 29 of the 64 cases. Delusional thinking of the perpetrator was noted in almost two-thirds of the "overkill" murders in this study.

Individuals admitted to a secure psychiatric hospital after committing parricide represent a unique subset of overall offenders. In a study by Baxter et al. (2001) reviewing 98 patients with mental disorders admitted to a secure hospital in England over 25 years who had killed their biological parents, the vast majority (approximately 91%) of perpetrators were men. Alcohol use was twice as likely in the stranger-killing group. The method of assault was similar across groups, with a sharp instrument being most common, followed by a blunt instrument, followed by strangulation. Firearms were rarely used (seen in only 6% of the parricide sample). This latter finding is understandable given the limited access to firearms in Great Britain. In a comparative study of news publications and reports searched in 2006 and published worldwide, 226 unique parricide incidents were reported (Boots and Heide 2006). From this study, 208 cases reported the type of weapon used. Firearms were used in 40%

of cases and knives in 21% of cases, with U.S. perpetrators more than twice as likely as perpetrators from non-U.S. countries to use firearms (49% vs 21%) and multiple weapons, whereas parricide killers from non-U.S. countries were significantly more likely than U.S. perpetrators to use knives (27% vs. 18%) and blunt objects (19% vs. 9%).

MOTIVATIONS

Walker (2016) found that the various rationales behind parricide in the sixteenth and seventeenth centuries revolved around themes of insanity, the outcome of parental abuse, and, most frequently, the sense that a child killing a parent was acting out of selfishness and seeing the parent as a barrier to desirable things such as riches, marriage, or other freedoms. This latter category highlighted moral and religious overtones linking the act of killing a parent to sinful conduct. From this viewpoint it logically flowed that the nature of the human condition was such that work was required to gain self-protection against becoming a sinner. Walker (2016) went on to state that by the eighteenth century, views that commission of parricide was a potential risk of the human condition shifted more toward the view that perpetrators were individually responsible for their actions.

Heide (1992) classified parricides on the basis of the type of perpetrator: the severely abused child, the severely mentally ill child, and the dangerously antisocial child. Subsequently, Hillbrand et al. (1999) categorized parricide on the basis of the age group of the perpetrators. Among youthful perpetrators, the authors noted child abuse, severe mental illness, budding antisocial personality disorder, and "precipitating factors" such as increasingly intolerable changes in circumstances. They cited Tanay's (1973) use of the term "reactive parricide" as one example of the type that derives from precipitating factors. It can include the culmination of tensions in a family of dysfunction. Among adult perpetrators of parricide, Hillbrand et al. affirmed that the majority struggle with severe mental illness but stressed that not all do. They therefore cautioned against leaping to the conclusion that mental illness is the ultimate cause, especially when there could be, regardless of mental illness, underlying family dynamics and dysfunction at play.

In consolidating the literature and examining 237 parricide cases committed by adult children, Hillbrand et al. (1999) found that more than three-quarters (79%) of offenders had some type of mood disorder or schizophrenia spectrum or other psychotic disorder. However, they observed that this finding represented an overestimate because of the generalities made regarding diagnoses in the original studies. They noted that the offender-victim relationships were often characterized by ongoing dependence of the adult offender and unemployment. Preexisting familial tensions were also noted. Hillbrand et al. observed that it is crucial to understand the nature of the relationship between the victim and the perpetrator and to not focus solely on any mental illness experienced by the perpetrator. In addition, nonpsychotic precursors identified included historical and perhaps long-standing abuse by the parent toward the child and sexual elements to the crime abuse or homicide.

Sadoff (1971) described two cases of patricide in-depth from a psychodynamic perspective and commented that the factor that seemed most striking to him was the "cruel and unusual relationship" between the parent and the son who killed him, including the intense ambivalence of hatred and longing as well as fear and loyalty.

Psychotic symptoms seen in the Hillbrand et al. (1999) case review included command hallucinations or delusional beliefs such as beliefs by the perpetrator that his or her parent had been replaced by an impostor, a witch, or even extraterrestrial beings. Green (1981) conducted a review of 58 cases in the United Kingdom and divided motives into paranoid persecutory beliefs, altruistic motivations, or other. Altruistic motives included murder as a means to end the suffering of the parent or to end the life of the parent when the perpetrator was dying and the parricide was an attempt to avoid the parent being left alone. Symptoms of mental illness such as depression were more commonly associated with this motivation for killings. A review of 27 U.S. parricide cases by Hillbrand et al. (1999) identified four subtypes: acute psychosis (47%), impulsive (28%), escape from enmeshment (15%), and alcohol or other substance use (seen in 24% of the cases) as a factor superimposed on the others.

As described earlier, Newhill (1991) delineated an alternative approach to categorizing parricide based on themes of family violence and available clinical information. She identified 17 factors that could be divided into three broad categories: 1) factors related to psychiatric status (e.g., the presence or absence of a diagnosable condition or symptoms); 2) factors related to interpersonal dynamics (e.g., the propensity for hostility, high emotionality, or violence in the home); and 3) demographics (characterized as whether the patient was a male under the age of 25).

UNIQUE ASSESSMENT ISSUES

The categorical schemes previously described (which undoubtedly are not exhausted by this listing) represent various ways to explain or understand parricide. Each one takes a slightly different approach from a different vantage point. On the basis of the various reported studies and reviews, an amalgamation of classification and typological schemes is warranted in trying to construct a framework for understanding these crimes. As noted, mental illness may or may not co-occur with several of the overarching typological constructs. From a review of the existing literature, the following categorical themes emerge, framed as questions for assessment and evaluation:

1. Was the act purposeful or nonpurposeful (including accidental)?
2. Was it impulsive or planned over time?
3. Was there an immediately precipitating event (e.g., such as an argument or substance use)?
4. What was the longer-term context of the preexisting dynamic (e.g., Were hostility and violence present in the family? Were there overcontrol issues in the dynamic? Was the parent suffering from end-of-life decline? Or was there no notable relevant preexisting family dynamic?)?
5. What was the motive (e.g., revenge against emotional, physical, or sexual child abuse, self-defense, profit or financial gain, achieving an outlet for anger, removal of parental control, achievement of some greater altruistic good, or the ability to gain sexual access to the parent)?
6. Did the perpetrator have a mental illness that could be linked to the crime or was it unrelated to the crime?
7. Did substance use play a role?
8. Were other nonparental victims involved that made the parricide only a portion of the event in question (e.g., family annihilation, serial killing, mass shootings)?

The examination of these factors can help construct a framework for what took place. Answers to these questions then will be able to guide treatment, intervention, and perhaps legal aftermath. Newhill (1991) also noted that the victim's role in family dynamic is important to consider—not to blame the victim, but to understand that these incidents of parricide may occur in the context of complex family dynamics in which the victim in some way precipitated the homicide (e.g., abuse, arguments, threats, belittling). For example, in the case of a substance-using child who gets into a fight with a parent and pushes him or her to his or her death, the death may have been "accidental" but precipitated by the problematic dynamics and a short-term impulsive action related to substance use. In the questions just laid out, the inquiry not only focuses on the actions and mental state of the perpetrator but considers these other background and intertwined aspects.

In any clinical or forensic assessment related to parricide, the means and the choice of weapon can provide further clues into the intensity and nature of the act (as noted earlier as whether there is an "overkill" context). For example, the use of a kitchen knife to stab a parent 100 times versus the use of a kitchen knife with one lethal stabbing; use of a family firearm versus the use of a firearm the perpetrator spent time acquiring just for this killing; or the acquisition and use of multiple firearms and assault weapons prior to the killing—all provide different snapshots into the circumstances.

LEGAL ISSUES

Most parricides are classified as murder (Boots and Heide 2006; Heide 1993b; Hillbrand et al. 1999), but there are different legal pathways for youthful and adult offenders. For youthful offenders, issues of child abuse might implicate defense strategies similar to battered wife syndrome (Bumby 1994). For adult offenders, Boots and Heide (2006) found that convictions were obtained in 93% of 226 media case reports reviewed for murder of various degrees, with about one-quarter of offenders being convicted on first-degree murder charges. Disposition of cases varied from a sentence of death (7%) to probation (6%). Life sentences without parole were seen most frequently (in 31% of the cases). Approximately 11% of offenders were ordered to go to a mental health facility, and 20% of case dispositions included an order for treatment. In the total cohort of 226 reports, overkill was seen in 20% of the cases (Boots and Heide 2006). Because these case reports were pulled from various media sources, this proportion of overkill cases may be an overrepresentation of the frequency of this phenomenon among all parricide incidents.

Parricide may evoke questions pertaining to the perpetrator's sanity at the time of the offense. In the study of individuals admitted to a secure psychiatric hospital in England, schizophrenia was the most common diagnosis among patients in the parricide group, and personality disorders were the most frequent diagnosis (with schizophrenia being a close second) for the patients who were admitted after killing a stranger (Baxter et al. 2001). The patients admitted to this psychiatric hospital, however, represent a limited sample of those who were already filtered through the criminal justice system and sent to a forensic hospital setting. Hillbrand et al. (1999) noted that insanity defenses for youth are rarely utilized.

Evaluations of criminal responsibility of those who have perpetrated parricide are not uncommon, although there is no formal study, to this author's knowledge, of data indicating the frequency of such evaluations. In conducting these evaluations, forensic examiners would follow the parameters in their particular state or jurisdiction, similar to the approach in other types of criminal evaluations. That said, understanding the individual family dynamics, factors related to domestic violence, and recognition of alternative strategies for coping with stress might help the examiner evaluate the perpetrator/defendant's abilities to know right from wrong or to appreciate the consequences of his or her actions. Shon and Roberts (2008) reviewed media reports from 100 crime scenes involving parricide in the late nineteenth century and found that postoffense behaviors could be categorized as ongoing violence, attempts at concealing the criminal act, or odd and unusual behaviors. Although this review reflected information on historic cases, the postcrime behavior can be informative in the consideration of an insanity defense.

For youths involved in a parricide, the potential for release at age 18 (or the relevant age at which juvenile jurisdiction terminates) is not at all implausible. Thus, provisions for postrelease supports with or without monitoring should be considered. The fact of the murder and the role of the perpetrator could be buried over time, given the protections often afforded in juvenile justice settings. In this author's experience, for example, a clinical consultation was sought for a woman, now in her 30s, who was receiving habilitative day services. She had killed a parent when she was 15 and was subsequently cared for by other family with no other history of violence known. Also, as seen in the case of the New Zealand girls who murdered one of their mothers, the girls were sent to juvenile facilities and then scattered to faraway locations.

In contrast to juveniles, the legal pathway for adults can vary much more between guilty findings and findings of not guilty by reason of insanity. Establishing the time frame to release (if release occurs) is not dependent on a finite age limit and thus can be more uncertain, especially if the perpetrator ends up in the forensic system.

AFTERMATH

Treatment of parricide offenders will depend on many factors, including the age of the perpetrators and the setting in which they are placed. If the perpetrator is a youth, he or she will most likely be placed within the confines of the juvenile justice setting. Within that setting, especially after adjudication, the youth would be able to avail himself or herself of whatever treatments are offered at that facility, although such facilities vary even in what type of treatment is available. Distress may manifest in suicidal thoughts and aggressive behavior, which might trigger a mental health response but could also trigger a response that leads to further isolation of the youth. A thorough assessment and evaluation of the youth at the outset is critical (Bumby 1994), not only to begin to understand the offense itself to help craft treatment but also to look at the emotional sequelae of the offensive act.

Myers (1992) articulated several factors for youths who have perpetrated homicide (whether parricide or not) and aptly noted the critical importance of time for further neurodevelopmental, cognitive, and emotional growth. Over time, a youth's sense of self, aggressive tendencies, and emotional state will evolve, making it even more important to conduct periodic assessments throughout a course of treatment. The intelligence of the youth, and his or her innate tendency toward aggression, can implicate or challenge the potential success of therapeutic interventions involving education and support (Myers 1992). In addition, the safety of the setting will be paramount to allow time to allow a healing process to begin, and efforts can be made to assist the youth toward a more positive adult outcome.

Regarding adult offenders, it is noteworthy that one Canadian study reviewed case data for 12 men who were thought to have a mental illness at the time of the parricide and found that almost half were reported to have sought psychiatric help in the several weeks before perpetrating the murder (Millaud et al. 1996). After the offense, treatment availability will vary, again, depending on setting. There are no specific treatments designed for adults who have perpetrated parricide. The usual array of services within a forensic hospital would include access to a multidisciplinary treatment team, therapy, and medications for treatable symptoms of mental illness, as well as activity and other active therapies that are available at the hospital. There will likely also be programming such as a gym or exercise that is offered and available as part of the rehabilitation during the time of "healing" from the events. Anger issues can be dealt with through various forms of cognitive-behavioral strategies. Medications should be used to help with symptoms such as psychosis or mood lability.

If the homicide was unrelated to mental illness and the offender ends up in a jail or prison, he or she will often be merged into the general population in that particular facility, although the offender might possibly be classified as "high risk." The criminal act may or may not be discussed overtly with anyone other than other inmates or correctional officers, and unless the offender avails himself or herself of psychiatric services, he or she could conceivably be left to cope with the incident—and the loss of the parent—without accessing any treatment or support. Even in cases in which the motive for parricide was to escape perceived abuse or complex dysfunctional family dynamics, ambivalence and confusion can be seen in the emotional aftermath of the killing. Some individuals may consider the death a relief, especially when parricide was motivated by years of abuse. Nevertheless, given the magnitude of this type of crime in our consciousness, it is likely that individual perpetrators could benefit from some type of therapeutic intervention including basic supportive therapy.

Family reconciliation may or may not be desired by the perpetrator or the remaining family but often emerges as an issue in therapy in the aftermath of the parricide. In this author's experience, the forgiveness of the child by a surviving parent can sometimes be an amazing dynamic to witness. Such forgiveness can arise in situations in which the parricide was seen as a rescue of the living parent from abuse. It can also be seen when there were other motives for the homicide. Forgiveness or lack thereof by siblings is equally unpredictable but may become part of the sequelae to sort through. When family reconciliation is desired, this should be done with the guidance of appropriate mental health practitioners who can help the family sort through ongoing issues and tensions as they arise.

The type of postrelease supervision, if any is assigned at all, will depend on whether the perpetrator was found guilty or not guilty by reason of insanity and the jurisdiction's rules about supervised release. In one study comparing mentally disordered parricide offenders and stranger killers who had been admitted to a maximum-security hospital in England after a mean of 6 years, neither group of patients committed a further homicide, and other rates of violence were low. In that particular study, the authors suggested that monitoring and placement restrictions of perpetrators might be higher than warranted by follow-up data (McCarthy et al. 2001). However, the authors also noted that there was no way to distinguish whether the low rate of violence postrelease was related to the supervision received or to the unique circumstances of the offense that were not later replicated.

In a study of cases of parricide committed between 1840 and 1899, some of the perpetrators went on to commit suicide after the killing (Seagrave 2009). In a more recent study of the mortality among Finnish male parricide offenders, one-third of deaths of all parricide offenders were the result of suicide, and rates of suicide were especially high for matricide offenders (Liettu et al. 2010). Interestingly also, the survival time after the offense was significantly shorter for males who committed matricide compared with those who committed other violence against a parent or patricide.

When suicide is contemporaneous with the parricide, the term *murder-suicide* may be used. When time and distance separates the suicide from the parricide, the suicide is considered a stand-alone issue. From the perspective of treatment, the individual who has committed a parricide should be considered at increased risk of suicide. Frequent assessments of overall risk of harm to self and others should be conducted, especially during a stabilization phase immediately after the parricide and while the individual is getting to know staff in a new placement such as a jail or psychiatric hospital. Ongoing risk assessment is needed because the act of killing one's parent will continue to be a chronic risk factor for suicide. Anniversary dates, birthdays, or holidays might worsen such risk. Thus, appropriate screening and monitoring should continue.

PREVENTION

A focus on prevention is always the best approach to avoid tragic outcomes. The difficulty lies, however, in developing prevention strategies when there are no recognized warning signs seen prospectively. That said, Millaud et al. (1996) noted that individuals who commit parricide might come to the attention of professionals prior to the murder, and as such there might be warnings potentially able to be known ahead of time. In other instances, within families there may be secrets that are not shared. An incestuous or abusive relationship, for example, may not come to light to those who can intervene. Abuse and violence can be multigenerational and considered "normal" for some families and there-fore would not naturally come to the attention of others unless child abuse is reported. Familial stressors can be numerous, and supports may be lacking. Cultural contexts may condone some violence, aggression, and limited rights, especially against youths or women. These factors can contribute to the risk of a fatal outcome. As noted, substance use or gen-eral aggression tolerance in a family can be other elements that raise risks within a family structure. Fascination with violence and weapons for some individuals may be part of the mix, as seen in the Newtown perpe-trator Adam Lanza, who killed his mother and then headed to an ele-mentary school to commit a mass shooting (Ziv 2014). In the Newtown case, the shooting motive was beyond parricide, but information emerged showing that Mr. Lanza's mother had increasingly worried about her son's mental state, including possible autism-like features, and she had difficulty accessing appropriate school services (Griffin and Kovner 2013). In the study by Bourget et al. (2007), there were several cases in which the victim had sought help and was in fear of his life prior to being killed but the concerns were not heeded.

The need for good risk assessment when an individual does come to the attention of a mental health professional cannot be overstated. Clini-cians should learn how to assess risks, including risk of harm to parents that might otherwise be overlooked, and they should obtain consultation. Because some of the motivations for parricide relate to chronic abuse, substance use in the home, and chronic familial dysfunction, prevention of these dynamics could help upstream prevention of a parricidal act where possible. Cases in which a son or daughter has developed a delu-sion involving a parent (e.g., paranoia that the parent means them harm or that the parent is a look-alike impostor [i.e., Capgras syndrome]) should raise red flags. In those instances, avoiding power and control struggles whenever possible might be prudent. For example, when an adult with mental illness and a paranoid delusion about their parents re-quires a guardian, it may be prudent to utilize a neutral party rather than a parent for the guardian's role. For parents of children who have been in-volved in stealing money or property for drugs, there could be cautionary safety planning set up for storage of cash and valuables. That said, parri-cide is rare and not a predictable phenomenon, meaning that in most cases these safeguards will not be necessary, and so an individual case-by-case determination and risk management will be important. General strategies of child abuse reporting, prevention of intrafamilial violence, and access to services are prevention strategies that can have potential for positive impact, even if their impact is not entirely measurable.

CONCLUSION

Parricide is thankfully a rare event. When it occurs, it generates media and larger societal interest and curiosity. Data on parricide are limited but demonstrate that incidents of parricide can stem from a variety of situations. Parricide by juveniles and parricide by adults reflect different phenomena. Serious mental illness is a relevant factor in a significant number of adult parricides, although not the majority. When serious mental illness is involved, typical symptoms include psychotic and mood symptoms. Extreme cases may include the phenomenon of overkill. The legal aftermath of the parricide will usually result in a conviction for murder, unless serious mental illness results in a finding of not guilty by reason of insanity. Treatment after the fact will vary depending on the age of the offender, his or her treatment needs, and the setting in which they are placed. Ongoing therapeutic approaches, risk assessment, and treatment of symptoms, including depression and suicidality, should occur for years after the incident. Although media reports and popular films depict these incidents with intrigue and high drama, when they occur, they leave devastation in their wake.

REFERENCES

Baxter H, Duggan C, Larkin E, et al: Mentally disordered parricide and stranger killers admitted to high-security care. 1: A descriptive comparison. The Journal of Forensic Psychiatry 12(2):287–299, 2001

Boots DP, Heide KM: Parricides in the media: a content analysis of available reports across cultures. Int J Offender Ther Comp Criminol 50(4):418–445, 2006 16837452

Bourget D, Gagné P, Labelle M-E: Parricide: a comparative study of matricide versus patricide. J Am Acad Psychiatry Law 35(3):306–312, 2007 17872550

Bumby KM: Psycholegal considerations in abuse-motivated parricides: children who kill their abusive parents. J Psychiatry Law 22(1):51–90, 1994

Davis D: Bad Blood: The Shocking True Story Behind the Menendez Killings. New York, St Martin's Press, 1994

Gillies A: The Parker-Hulme murder: why it still matters to us. New Zealand Herald, November 14, 2011. Available at: http://www.nzherald.co.nz/nz/news/article.cfm?c_id=1&objectid=10765998. Accessed February 2, 2017.

Green CM: Matricide by sons. Med Sci Law 21(3):207–214, 1981 7278533

Griffin A, Kovner J: Adam Lanza's medical records reveal growing anxiety. Hartford Courant, June 20, 2013. Available at: http://www.courant.com/news/connecticut/newtown-sandy-hook-school-shooting/hc-adam-lanza-pediatric-records-20130629,0,7137229.story. Accessed June 14, 2017.

Heide KM: Why Kids Kill Parents: Child Abuse and Adolescent Homicide. Columbus, Ohio State University Press, 1992

Heide KM: Parents who get killed and the children who kill them. J Interpers Violence 8(4):531–544, 1993a

Heide KM: Weapons used by juveniles and adults to kill parents. Behav Sci Law 11(4):397–405, 1993b

Heide KM, Petee TA: Parricide: an empirical analysis of 24 years of U.S. data. J Interpers Violence 22(11):1382–1399, 2007 17925288

Hillbrand M, Alexandre JW, Young JL, et al: Parricides: characteristics of offenders and victims, legal factors, and treatment issues. Aggress Violent Behav 4(2):179–190, 1999

Liettu A, Mikkola L, Säävälä H, et al: Mortality rates of males who commit parricide or other violent offense against a parent. J Am Acad Psychiatry Law 38(2):212–220, 2010 20542941

McCarthy L, Page K, Baxter H, et al: Mentally disordered parricide and stranger killers admitted to high-security care. 2: Course after release. The Journal of Forensic Psychiatry 12(3):501–514, 2001

Menendez v Superior Court, Supreme Court of California, 834 P.2d 786, (1992)

Millaud F, Auclair N, Meunier D: Parricide and mental illness. A study of 12 cases. Int J Law Psychiatry 19(2):173–182, 1996 8725654

Myers WC: What treatments do we have for children and adolescents who have killed? Bull Am Acad Psychiatry Law 20(1):47–58, 1992 1576375

Newhill CE: Parricide. J Fam Violence 6(4):375–394, 1991

Parker P: Diaries. The Heavenly Creatures Website, 2014. Available at: http://www.adamabrams.com/hc/faq2/Section_7/7.4.3.html. Accessed November 20, 2017.

Sadoff RL: Clinical observations on parricide. Psychiatr Q 45(1):65–69, 1971 5120053

Seagrave K: Parricide in the United States: 1840–1899. Jefferson, NC, McFarland & Co, 2009

Shon PC, Roberts MA: Post-offence characteristics of 19th-century American parricides: an archival exploration. Journal of Investigative Psychology and Offender Profiling 5(3):147–169, 2008

Shon PCH, Targonski JR: Declining trends in U.S. parricides, 1976–1998: testing the Freudian assumptions. Int J Law Psychiatry 26(4):387–402, 2003 12726812

Stoessel T, Bornstein SJ: Enquête sur le parricide en France en 1985 et 1986. Annales de Psychiatrique 3(3):222–229, 1988

Tanay E: Proceedings: adolescents who kill parents—reactive parricide. Aust N Z J Psychiatry 7(4):263–277, 1973 4522943

Walker G: Imagining the unimaginable: parricide in early modern England and Wales, c. 1600–c. 1760. J Fam Hist 41(3):271–293, 2016 27365565

Walsh JA, Krienert JL, Crowder D: Innocence lost: a gender-based study of parricide offender, victim, and incident characteristics in a national sample, 1976–2003. J Aggress Maltreat Trauma 16(2):202–227, 2008

Ziv S: Report details Adam Lanza's life before Sandy Hook shootings. Newsweek, November 25, 2014. Available at: http://www.newsweek.com/report-details-adam-lanzas-life-sandy-hook-shootings-286867. Accessed November 12, 2017.

9

Intimate Partner Homicide in Elderly Populations

Jacob M. Appel, M.D., J.D., M.P.H.

INTRODUCTION: "A GERIATRIC ROMEO AND JULIET"

On January 19, 2014, 88-year-old William Dresser walked into a hospital room at Carson Tahoe Regional Medical Center in Nevada and shot his 86-year-old wife, Frances, in the chest with a .22 caliber pistol (Marcus 2014). Before Dresser could turn the weapon on himself—he later told investigators he had four bullets, two for each of them—the gun jammed and broke apart in his hands. Moments later, the elderly man was detained by security officers and jailed on a murder charge. He later explained his motive to the *Reno Gazette-Journal* with clarity: "The fact [was] that she had no future and was miserable and begging to die" (Marcus 2014). His wife had fallen at home several weeks earlier; she remained unable to move her limbs and was in intractable pain. As her distraught husband saw it, "[S]he was paralyzed from the neck down and very uncomfortable without much of a future, so I just helped her along" (Marcus 2014). The pair had been married for 63 years.

William Dresser was, at first glance, an unlikely killer. By all accounts a devoted husband and father to three adult children, William was—in the words of his daughter, Kelly Dresser LeCount—"a stellar human being" (Gardner 2014). "Since they met, they were joined at the hip," she told the *Nevada Appeal*. "He was a mail carrier, and she was a pretty girl he saw sunbathing in a neighbor's yard" (Gardner 2014). In the days leading up to Frances's death, LeCount's family had been attempting to bring her paralyzed mother home for hospice care. Yet, according to William, his wife asked him directly and repeatedly to end her suffering. "I think Mommy and Daddy saw this as a way out of their broken, hurting bodies and on the road to their next adventure," LeCount reflected (Gardner 2014). She described her parents as a "geriatric Romeo and Juliet" (Gardner 2014). At the time of the killing, William was himself battling cancer. "Why would you hold [the killing] against a man who was so damn near perfect?" asked LeCount (Gardner 2014). "I can't imagine my dad is too long for this world.... I would like it if he could enjoy his last few days at home."

Carson City District Attorney Jason Woodbury eventually agreed with the Dresser family, none of whom reportedly blamed William for his actions. Eighteen months after William was released on bail, Woodbury formally dropped all charges against him. "I didn't view there being any component of evil to his act of killing," the prosecutor explained to the media. "We can talk about judgment—and morally whether it was a right or wrong decision—but I didn't view any aspect of it as evil. That's truly the component you need to have in a murder case—an evil motive—and we didn't have that" (Pickles 2015). Carson City Sheriff Kenneth Furlong supported this controversial decision. "I don't condone what [Dresser] did whatsoever, whatsoever," he said, "[This is] a real challenge for our system.... You can't condone the behavior, but what do you do with it once the behavior occurs?" (Damon 2015a, 2015b). According to the *Nevada Appeal,* another factor in the choice not to prosecute was a potential trial's $200,000 price tag and, if Dresser were jailed, an additional $72,000–$96,000 liability for his medication costs (Pettaway 2015). The case prompted Democratic State Senator David Parks to introduce a "death with dignity" bill before Nevada's state legislature (Marcus 2014). "[H]aving this avenue would certainly avoid doing a murder-suicide....a horrible thing we hear on a regular basis," he said (Marcus 2014), although the claim that aid-in-dying legislation will reduce intimate partner killings among the elderly remains highly controversial.

Although William Dresser did not meet society's expectations for the image of a killer, high-profile cases like his are growing increasingly frequent. Media reports of murder-suicides and so-called "mercy killings" among the elderly have become so commonplace, in fact, and these acts have been tolerated so often, that a *Huffington Post* headline posed the provocative question: "Elderly Murder-Suicide: Should We Praise Old Men Who Kill Their Wives and Themselves?" (Marquardt 2012). Answers vary widely among health care professionals, policymakers, and the families of the victims.

OVERVIEW

Data on homicide in elderly populations are relatively scarce (Bourget et al. 2010). Among the factors that have historically limited such research are the comparative infrequency of killings among older populations; the increased likelihood that these killings will occur between intimate partners, reducing the danger to the general public; and a belief, at least in some quarters, that so-called mercy killings among the elderly are justifiable, if unfortunate, in the absence of better elder care and assisted suicide legislation. Murder-suicides constitute a considerable percentage of these killings and are among the most studied. What data do exist often come from the study of media reports and high-profile cases, which may not reflect overall patterns of behavior.

Homicides among the elderly appear to fit conceptually into three broad categories, although significant overlap likely exists between these groups; in fact, one might consider these three groups as existing on a trilateral continuum where discrete classification is often difficult and hybrids constitute the vast majority of cases.

The first category of killings occurs in the domestic setting between spouses or intimate partners established in long-term, stable, and previously positive relationships—such as the marriage of the Dressers, as described. One of the partners becomes ill, or both partners face deteriorations in health. What follows is a so-called mercy killing or mercy killing followed by suicide, in which one spouse, predominantly the husband, ends the life of the partner with the purported intent of preserving dignity and terminating suffering. Some of these killings occur with the explicit consent of—or even at the behest of—the victim. However, such overt agreements between partners appear to be rare (4%; Salari 2007). Other incidents result from the vicarious assessment by the perpetrator of what the victim would have wanted, although sometimes these assessments prove wrong. Often these episodes are portrayed sympathetically in the media, as was the killing of Frances Dresser, and brought up in the context of the ongoing debate over legalized aid-in-dying for the terminally ill.

A second related but possibly distinct set of killings are those in which suicide of the perpetrator is the primary or original intent and the killing of the spouse arises secondarily—as an afterthought, one might say. As described by one researcher, "[T]he typical situation involved a perpetrator who planned to kill him/herself, but at some point prior to the act, made the decision to kill their partner. They may have been concerned about how the spouse would handle the suicide. Another possibility is that they viewed their spouse as an extension of themselves, rather than an autonomous person" (Salari 2007, p. 155). Both physical and psychiatric illnesses are among the likely forces driving the initial interest in suicide (Reese 2013; Rosenbaum 1990). Substance abuse plays a role in some cases, as do social isolation and financial setbacks. One large study reported that in intimate elderly homicide cases, only the perpetrator, and not the victim, was ill in a striking 30% of cases (Salari 2007).

A third category of killings reflects an escalation of ongoing or long-standing intimate partner violence (Roberto et al. 2013b). One study documented a known history of domestic violence in 14% of cases, with 12% of perpetrators qualifying as "intimate terrorists" who had engaged in "threats, violence, and other power and control tactics to severely isolate the victim" prior to the killing (Salari 2007, p. 443). Secondary victims, such as other relatives, may also be killed or injured in such incidents (Salari 2007), although one should recognize that third parties may also be killed or injured inadvertently during classic "mercy killings," as in a high-profile Houston, Texas, case in which a son was shot trying to break up his parents' murder-suicide (Hinchliffe 2015). Some evidence exists that a "suicide contagion" effect occurs, with murder-suicides among the elderly leading to "copycat" offenses (Salari 2007).

Critics of these distinctions suggest that searching for dividing lines between "mercy killings," murders secondary to suicides, and escalations of intimate partner violence may prove misleading. As one scholar noted, "Relatively harmless gender norms (e.g., loving husband as family decision-maker) may have extreme consequences later in life, as older men make decisions under the stress of caregiving. If a husband is not in the habit of considering his wife's autonomy, he may use an extreme approach to take control of the situation, such as murder, to deal with her perceived suffering and his increasing care burden" (Roberto et al. 2013a, p. 237). Some critics argue that viewing any of these killings through the lens of "mercy" is misguided; rather, they see genuine "mercy killings" as exceedingly rare and "[l]ater life intimate partner homicide suicide" as representing "the most severe form of domestic partner abuse" (Salari 2007, p. 441).

Suicide pacts in which two elderly persons in an intimate relationship kill themselves simultaneously, or in close succession, also merit examination. This phenomenon gained significant notice in 2002, when 86-year-old naval hero Chester W. Nimitz Jr. and his wife, Joan, age 89, overdosed on sleeping pills as part of a mutual suicide pact (Rimer 2002). Some of these cases may reflect those same factors that underlie suicide more generally. However, in others, one party may be acting under significant emotional duress. When joint suicides reflect the extreme pressure of one party upon another, especially in the setting of a long-term intimate or familiar relationship, the distinction between mutual suicide and murder-suicide weakens. Yet because these tragedies generally occur in private, investigators can rarely be confident that one of the parties did not act under duress. None of the safeguards built into legalized aid-in-dying, such as the laws in the six states where assisted suicide is now legal (Oregon, Washington, Montana, Vermont, California, and Colorado), exist when individuals pursue their ends extralegally. For example, in the absence of a psychiatric examination, one cannot discern the victim's state of mind prior to death—not only whether she sought aid-in-dying but also whether she had the capacity to make such a choice. The hazy boundary between murder-suicide and joint suicide under duress further complicates obtaining meaningful data on the subject.

Bias may exist in the presentation of these cases to the public. Journalist and media outlets sympathetic to assisted suicide for the terminally ill may be more willing to publicize cases in which both parties sought death over those involving intimate partner violence. Similarly, families may prove more willing to discuss their deceased relatives, as did Kelly Dresser LeCount, when the motives of the perpetrator seem altruistic rather than disturbed. This bias may distort public perceptions of the underlying issues, distract providers from appropriate preventive measures, and prove challenging to researchers seeking to expand knowledge is this area.

EPIDEMIOLOGY

In contrast to homicides involving younger killers, "most homicides committed by offenders aged 65 and older occur in a domestic context"

(Bourget et al. 2010, p. 305). The frequency of these episodes varies considerably across nations and cultures, but the incidence in North America is increasing. The Violence Policy Center reported that murder-suicides among those older than 55 years in the United States increased from 21% of all murder-suicides in 2002 to 25% in 2011 (Reese 2013). Rates are increasing in Canada as well (Bourget et al. 2010). This development contrasts with an overall murder-suicide rate that remains relatively low and stable (Eliason 2009). Unfortunately, elderly-upon-elderly killing has been significantly understudied, and the limited empirical data are often contradictory. The most comprehensive data appear to be found in Cohen et al.'s (1998) study of seven Florida counties between 1988 and 1994 and in Salari's (2007) study of homicide-suicide in the elderly, but the degree to which these data may be generalizable remains uncertain. Complicating matters further are the significant regional differences found by Cohen et al. (1998)—even within the state of Florida—a geographic variation that was not found among younger killers. Although rare, homicides and murder-suicides among the elderly do appear to have features that distinguish them from similar phenomena in younger age groups (Eliason 2009).

One consistent feature of these killings is that the perpetrators appear overwhelmingly to be male and the victims to be female. This male predominance is present in all murder-suicides but is increasingly so among those older than 55 years (Cohen et al. 1998). Salari (2007) found that in homicide-suicide cases, 96% of the perpetrators were male. In the United States, male perpetrators tend to be older, often considerably so, than their spouses (Bourget et al. 2010), whereas in Canada, 77% of perpetrators were close in age to their victims (Bourget et al. 2010).

Firearms were the most common method used (Salari 2007). The majority of such killings occurred in the home, rather than in institutions or in public settings (Salari 2007).

A history of domestic violence remains a significant risk factor for spousal killings in elderly populations (Bourget et al. 2010), but the prevalence of intimate partner violence prior to such killings is uncertain. Salari (2007) found such conflict to be a factor in approximately one-third of homicide-suicides in this age group. Although "relationship strife was present in some cases," the rate was only "slightly higher than the divorce rate for that age group" (Salari 2007, p. 441). Cohen et al. (1998) found physical violence to be "prominent" in between 4% and 14% of cases, depending on the county. Recent legal difficulties and criminal complaints may also be a factor, although the prevalence again varied geographically (Cohen et al. 1998).

Physical illness frequently appears to be a contributing factor in such cases, affecting either the perpetrator, the victim, or both partners (Bourget et al. 2010). Significant declines in physical health, whether actual or perceived, occurred in many couples (Cohen 2000). The threat of separation contributed significantly to risk, as a spouse facing relocation to a long-term care facility was at particularly increased jeopardy (Bourget et al. 2010). The husband was "caregiver for a wife with a longstanding disabling or terminal chronic illness" in a sizable percentage of cases, and many men reported feeling unable to care for their wives (Bourget et al. 2010, p. 306).

The degree to which mental illness and/or substance abuse contribute to these killings is more controversial, but they clearly play a significant role in some cases. Bourget et al. (2010) argued that "[m]ost of the men" have "untreated depression or another undiagnosed mental illness" (p. 306). Cohen et al. (1998) found that "[i]n west central Florida, the following features were identified in the medical examiner records of the older perpetrators: 37% were depressed, 11% were abusing alcohol or drugs, 15% had talked about suicide, and 4% had previously attempted suicide" (p. 393), while "[i]n southeastern Florida depression was described for 19% of the older perpetrators, other mental illness in 10%, and talk of suicide in 24%" (p. 393). (Explanations for these differences between regions include the racial/ethnic makeup of the counties—most of the west central Florida couples were white, whereas most of those in southeast Florida were Hispanic—as well as marital status, health status, and old age vs. very old age.) These findings correlate with data from the general population showing that mental illness contributes significantly to overall murder-suicide rates and that pathology may also play a role (Rosenbaum 1990). For those whose underlying motive is suicide, depression certainly appears likely to play a contributory role (Salari 2007). Salari (2007) found minimal evidence for "major psychotic pathology" or "the influence of substances" such as alcohol and illicit drugs in elderly homicide-suicide cases. In contrast, Cohen et al. (1998) did find alcohol to be a factor in up to half of such deaths.

The role of dementia in elderly spousal killings and homicide-suicides remains controversial. Although Alzheimer's disease was previously thought to increase the risk to both the sufferer and spouse, possibly through increased caregiver burden, Malphurs et al. (2001) found that a diagnosis of Alzheimer's disease only increases a caregiver's risk of dying by suicide, not committing homicide. The authors argued this finding is "consistent with the interpretation that planning and executing a homicide-suicide is cognitively more complex than planning and carrying out a suicide" (Malphurs et al. 2001, p. 55). Similarly, Salari (2007) found no significant role for Alzheimer's disease in homicide-suicide cases.

MOTIVATIONS

Why do elderly spouses kill their partners? One helpful approach is to distinguish "altruistic" motivation homicides (Marzuk et al. 1992) from "egotistic" motivation killings (Salari 2007). In the former, the perpetrator is driven to help someone other than himself—often either to terminate the suffering of his partner or to reduce the care burden in his family. He may conceive of the former case as "doing the victim a favor" (Salari 2007). Obviously, these motives may not reflect the actual wishes of the victim or of family members, but the perpetrator—rightly or wrongly—perceives himself as serving outside interests. In contrast, "egotistic" killings are driven largely by the welfare of the perpetrator himself: this may include the personal desire to escape his role as a caregiver, emotional or financial strain, or the urge to assert control in a setting in which his own illness or disability has rendered him compromised. Many male spouses, particularly those of a controlling nature or chronic perpetrators of abuse, may simply not wish their wives to continue living beyond their own deaths. Some "egotistic" perpetrators may, of course, convince themselves that they are acting out of altruistic motives; others may simply use altruistic arguments as defenses if they survive a homicide-suicide attempt or never intended contemporaneous suicide. Unscrupulous perpetrators may, on rare occasions, even seek to disguise old-fashioned homicides, such as those motivated by jealousy or pecuniary gain, as mercy killings.

LEGAL DISPOSITION AND CONSEQUENCES

Many intimate homicides between the elderly are homicide-suicides, or attempted homicide-suicides, so often cases have no legal sequelae. Survival rates of the perpetrating partner in such attempts tend be extremely low; a retrospective study of 225 such events found at least one survivor in only 22 instances (Salari 2007). Those who survive can often find themselves severely injured or impaired through their attempts, further reducing the number of cases involving elderly partners that actually lead to prosecution.

Concrete data on prosecution rates are not available at this time. However, anecdotal evidence strongly suggests that many cases of intimate homicide among the elderly do not lead to prosecution. Perpetrators may be too physically ill or too psychologically vulnerable to stand trial—with prosecutors exercising wide leeway not to pursue such cases. Public sympathy, whether reasonably or not, often sides with the killer. Few district attorneys wish to be seen prosecuting elderly spouses in alleged "mercy killings" when doing so runs against popular opinion. In many cases, such as that of the Dressers, adult children and other family members advocate strongly against criminal charges. Finally, the length of the judicial process likely prevents some perpetrators, already old and ill, from surviving long enough to face a judge.

Spousal murders among the elderly have consequences that transcend perpetrator and victim. As Salari (2007) noted of elderly homicide-suicides, these tragedies have "far reaching effects on public health as events traumatize families, friends, neighborhoods and entire communities" (p. 441). The violent death of a close relative, even when genuinely perpetrated with altruistic intent, cannot be without significant emotional consequences for survivors. The survivors are often denied both an opportunity to say farewell to their loved ones and their proverbial day in court. In short, these extralegal killings are socially disruptive events and tear at our societal fabric.

PREVENTION

The first question to ask regarding the prevention of intimate partner killing among the elderly is whether universal prevention is actually desirable—or whether, under limited circumstances, such killings should be tolerated. Assuming the three-category framework discussed earlier has some validity, one suspects that reasonable people could easily reach a consensus on the desirability of preventing the killings described in the second and third category—those in which the perpetrator acts secondary to suicidal intent or as a culmination of ongoing intimate partner violence. However, when one considers genuine "mercy killings," as described in the first category, that occur in jurisdictions where aid-in-dying or assisted suicide remains illegal, considerable disagreement likely exists as to whether such killings ought to be prevented. Some ethicists argue that extralegal "mercy killing" is justified in the absence of legal sanction—and that preventing such killings is not inherently desirable. Others, of course, disagree. Yet given the choice between legal and extralegal killings, a strong argument exists for the establishment of a legal and regulated system for aid-in-dying that ensures safeguards for autonomy that cannot be assured outside the law.

It is worth noting that many of the leading authors in this field come to the subject of intimate partner homicide among the elderly from backgrounds of research or activism in which they sought to mitigate intimate partner violence, leading them to emphasize universal prevention. In contrast, advocates for aid-in-dying for the elderly focus on so-called mercy killing cases and rarely write about preventing homicides stemming from suicidality or intimate partner violence. No conclusive data yet exist on whether assisted-suicide legalization reduces rates of intimate partner homicide in the elderly. This author takes no normative stand on the issue in this chapter. Rather, what follows is a discussion of prevention methods that may be applied in cases in which they are deemed to be desirable.

Interventions specifically to prevent spousal murder among the elderly have generally not yet been studied. Most authorities recommend similar interventions that are used to address either the underlying causes of such killings in the general population, such as intimate partner violence, or suicide among the elderly, including depression and caregiver burnout. Malphurs et al. (2001) argued for early interventions that use a careful assessment of risk and protective factors. Increasing social supports for elderly caregivers, especially male caregivers, seems essential. Reductions in firearms ownership by vulnerable individuals in these households might also prove beneficial. Finally, Malphurs et al. contend that "substantial efforts are needed to increase the knowledge of primary care physicians, other professionals, and families about the detection and appropriate treatment of depression and marital stress in older men and their wives" (p. 56). At present, both providers and the public generally know little about such killings beyond the nonrepresentative cases reported in the media; this limited-awareness, distorted perception likely leads to reduced screening and ultimately more deaths.

Complicating any efforts at prevention are specific factors that are related to "gender socialization and the use of formal services" that apply particularly to current cohorts of senior citizens (Salari 2007). Our current elderly population came of age at a time when mental illness was stigmatized and domestic abuse was considered a private matter (Salari 2007). Gender norms relating to male authority and control, alien to many young people today, can still be found among elderly couples, further contributing to the challenge faced by those seeking to prevent such killings (Salari and Zhang 2006).

CONCLUSION

The tragedy of William and Frances Dresser reflects many of the ongoing challenges that the medical and legal systems confront in cases of elderly spousal homicide. In some regard, the details are paradigmatic: William was the male partner, both spouses suffered from significant disabilities, and a firearm proved the weapon of choice. Other features of the killing seem atypical. There appears to be some concrete evidence that Frances expressed a wish to die; William's family members seem to have been actively engaged in their parents' care; no evidence of domestic abuse or violence came to the surface during an extensive investigation. Some crucial questions remain unanswered—and possibly unanswerable: Was William motivated by his own increasing frailty or solely by his wife's? Were his motives altruistic, egotistical, or some combination of both? Cases like that of the Dressers reveal the substantial and inevitable uncertainties that arise when such killings occur outside of legal sanction and regulation. We may simply never know with any confidence what brought a marriage of 63 years to an end in an act of extreme violence.

REFERENCES

Bourget D, Gagné P, Whitehurst L: Domestic homicide and homicide-suicide: the older offender. J Am Acad Psychiatry Law 38(3):305–311, 2010 20852214

Cohen D: Homicide-suicide in older persons. Psychiatr Times 17:49–52, 2000

Cohen D, Llorente M, Eisdorfer C: Homicide-suicide in older persons. Am J Psychiatry 155(3):390–396, 1998 9501751

Damon A: DA seeks to drop mercy-killing murder charge in Nevada. Reno Gazette Journal, June 19, 2015a. Available at: http://www.usatoday.com/story/news/nation/2015/06/19/da-seeks-drop-mercy-killing-murder-charge-nevada/29019813/. Accessed April 14, 2016.

Damon A: 'No evil in his act': DA seeks to drop mercy killing murder charge. Reno Gazette Journal, June 22, 2015b. Available at: http://www.rgj.com/story/news/2015/06/19/evil-act-da-seeks-drop-mercy-killing-murder-charge/29006263/. Accessed April 14, 2016.

Eliason S: Murder-suicide: a review of the recent literature. J Am Acad Psychiatry Law 37(3):371–376, 2009 19767502

Gardner S: 'Their final, great act of love.' Nevada Appeal, January 31, 2014. Available at: http://www.nevadaappeal.com/news/local/their-final-great-act-of-love/. Accessed April 14, 2016.

Hinchliffe E: Son injured trying to break up father's murder-suicide. Houston Chronicle, November 4, 2015

Malphurs JE, Eisdorfer C, Cohen D: A comparison of antecedents of homicide-suicide and suicide in older married men. Am J Geriatr Psychiatry 9(1):49–57, 2001 11156752

Marcus E: Shooting suspect says ailing wife 'begging to die.' Reno Gazette Journal, January 29, 2014. Available at: http://www.usatoday.com/story/news/nation/2014/01/29/shooting-suspect-says-ailing-wife-begging-to-die-/5040877/. Accessed April 14, 2016.

Marquardt E: Elderly murder-suicide: should we praise old men who kill their wives and themselves? Huffington Post, June 9, 2012. Available at: http://www.huffingtonpost.com/elizabeth-marquardt/elderly-murder-suicide_b_1402935.html. Accessed April 14, 2016.

Marzuk PM, Tardiff K, Hirsch CS: The epidemiology of murder-suicide. JAMA 267(23):3179–3183, 1992 1593740

Pettaway T: Carson City district attorney dismisses William Dresser murder charges. Nevada Appeal, June 18, 2015

Pickles K: 'No evil in his act': DA seeks to drop murder charge against 88-year-old who shot his paralyzed wife, 86, in 'mercy killing.' The Daily Mail (United Kingdom), June 22, 2015. Available at: http://www.dailymail.co.uk/news/article-3134424/No-evil-act-DA-seeks-drop-mercy-killing-murder-charge-against-88-year-old-man-shot-paralyzed-86-year-old-wife.html. Accessed April 14, 2016.

Reese D: Murder-suicide disturbing trend among elderly. The Washington Post, January 26, 2013

Rimer S: With suicide, an Admiral keeps command until the end. The New York Times, January 12, 2002

Roberto KA, McCann BR, Brossoie N: Intimate partner violence in late life: an analysis of national news reports. J Elder Abuse Negl 25(3):230–241, 2013a 23627429

Roberto KA, McPherson MC, Brossoie N: Intimate partner violence in late life: a review of the empirical literature. Violence Against Women 19(12):1538–1558, 2013b 24476758

Rosenbaum M: The role of depression in couples involved in murder-suicide and homicide. Am J Psychiatry 147(8):1036–1039, 1990 2375438

Salari S: Patterns of intimate partner homicide suicide in later life: strategies for prevention. Clin Interv Aging 2(3):441–452, 2007 18044194

Salari S, Zhang W: Kin keepers and good providers: influence of gender socialization on well-being among USA birth cohorts. Aging Ment Health 10(5):485–496, 2006 16938684

10

Familicide

Family Annihilation

Richard Martinez, M.D., M.H.

INTRODUCTION

On September 10, 2015, Sergeant Jim Williams with the South Lake Minnetonka Police Department was sent to the home of Brian Short after a 911 caller stated that Mr. Short, age 45, had not shown up for work for several days and that his three children—Cole, age 17; Madison, age 15; and Brooklyn, age 14—had not attended school. The caller, Mr. Short's coworker, had told police that Brian had recently inquired about life insurance policies and the suicide clause in the benefits. Investigation would later reveal that the children's school began a new year on September 8, and the children had not come to school for the 2 days prior to when Sgt. Williams was sent to the home to investigate. As Sgt. Williams entered the unlocked back door of the Short's $2 million mansion in Greenwood, Minnesota, shortly after the lunch hour, he was apprehensive, as he quickly realized this was not a typical welfare check.

Upon entering the home, Sgt. Williams found the body of Mr. Short's wife, Karen, in her bedroom. "Horrific," Sgt. Williams was quoted several months after the tragedy. "It was the worst thing I've ever seen." As he went through the home, he discovered the bodies of the three children and found the body of Brian Short in the garage. All deaths were due to gunshots from a shotgun at close range, allegedly fired by Mr. Short. Investigators discovered that Mr. Short, a former nurse who had created and developed a successful social media website, AllNurses.com, 20 years earlier, was facing financial stress, including a defamation lawsuit against his company. Teenagers from the children's high school reported that one of the children mentioned they would be selling their 5,600-square foot home for something smaller, and another report revealed the family had recently ended weekly cleaning services. Mr. Short had entered mental health treatment and was receiving medication. According to a neighbor, days before the shooting, Mr. Short had made a gesture by placing his hand in the shape of a gun to his head and stating, "It's just overwhelming" (Kieffer 2016).

OVERVIEW

Familicide is the type of murder or murder-suicide wherein members of a family are killed in quick succession, followed in some cases by the suicide of the perpetrator. In these multiple-victim homicides, it is the killer's spouse, ex-spouse, or partner and commonly one or more children who are killed (Wilson et al. 1995), although cases in which children murder their parents and siblings are also termed familicides. In the vast majority of cases, the killer is the father. In some cases, in addition to a spouse and children, other relatives, such as the aggressor's parents or siblings, are killed. In tragedies where all members of the family are killed followed by the suicide of the person who committed the murders, the crime is labeled "family annihilation" (Dietz 1986). Although these murders are classified as mass murders, they usually involve the killing of loved ones and not strangers. However, a variety of this category of homicide can include mass murderers who first kill family members and then murder strangers. In general, familicide and family annihilations can be understood as phenomena that share characteristics with filicide-suicides (i.e., killing children prior to suicide), which do not include the murder of a spouse. Resnick's (1969) early article offering a phenomenological typology based on the killer's motives is useful in looking at this category of homicide (Hatters Friedman et al. 2005). In Resnick's early work, he characterized filicides as 1) altruistic, 2) acutely psychotic, 3) accidental (fatal maltreatment), 4) due to an unwanted child, and 5) spouse revenge (see Chapter 6).

Charles Whitman, the University of Texas tower sniper, is one of the most notorious variations on the family annihilation phenomena. Whitman first killed his wife and mother, then went to the tower of the main building on the University of Texas at Austin campus and killed 14 more people (Newberger 2016). Familicides are rare; however, these events are usually reacted to with understandable horror. It is often the case that relatives and friends describe feeling shocked, sometimes stating that there was nothing in their experience with the killer to suggest that such violence was possible. Often the family is described as appearing to be loving and without obvious evidence of domestic turmoil, which is one of the reasons that these tragedies are so disturbing to surviving relatives and friends. In the media, these killings are often characterized as lacking warning signs, with the killer exhibiting no prior public behaviors that would allow for intervention or prevention of the tragedy. In addition, although not with Charles Whitman, these cases usually involve the murder of children, which is counter to expectations of parental protection and nurturance. For most people, this makes it difficult to empathize with the perpetrator of these acts.

As a subcategory of mass murder, familicides account for more than half of those killed in mass murders (Duwe 2004, 2007). Therefore, this is the most common form of mass killings in the United States, in spite of the misperception promoted by media reports in recent years of mass killings involving terrorism. Because these mass murders involve intimate relationships within families, the psychological aspect of these murders is much different than the psychological aspect of the mass murders in which individuals kill large numbers of strangers. Although there are prominent and disturbing attacks in public spaces such as the Orlando Pulse nightclub attack in 2016 and the San Bernardino Inland Regional Center shooting in 2015, the vast majority of mass killings occur in the home, and the majority involve the killing of family and relatives. Similar to other mass killings, these familicides usually occur in a single location and typically in a short time frame.

EPIDEMIOLOGY

Although the Centers for Disease Control and Prevention's National Violent Death Reporting System collects data from law enforcement, medical examiners, vital statistics, and crime laboratories, actual statistics on this type of murder are limited. Familicides, along with other mass killings, including serial and spree killings (Morton and Hilts 2005), account for less than 0.1% of the roughly 20,000 homicides each year in the United States (Duwe 2004, 2007). One method of conceptualizing these tragedies in which the killer commits suicide is as a subset of murder-suicide. The Violence Policy Center, a nonprofit educational organization that conducts research and promotes public education on violence in America, has collected information on murder-suicides since 2002 and published their information in a fifth edition in 2015 (Violence Policy Center 2015).

In the Violence Policy Center's estimate, in the first half of 2014 in the United States, there were 285 murder-suicide events resulting in 617 murder-suicide deaths, of which 285 were suicides and 332 homicides. Of the 285 perpetrators who committed suicide, 254 were male and 30 were female. In their study of the 332 homicides, 252 victims were female and 79 victims were male; 45 of the homicide victims were children and teenagers younger than 18 years. Sixty-three children and teens younger than 18 years survived and witnessed some aspect of the murder-suicide. Almost three-quarters (72%) of all murder-suicides involved an intimate partner. Of these, 93% were females killed by their intimate partners. Of the total murder-suicide events for the 6-month period, 93% involved the use of a firearm. The Violence Policy Center extrapolated that on average there were 11 murder-suicide events each week, and there were 1,234 murder-suicide deaths in 2014. Because much of this information was obtained by tracking news reports across the United States, the researchers believe this to be an underestimate (Violence Policy Center 2015).

Additional information from the Violence Policy Center study in 2015 showed that 89% of the offenders were males acting alone. This is supported by other studies in the United States that have shown that 90% of murder-suicides involve male perpetrators (Auchter 2010; Felthous and Hempel 1995; Marzuk et al. 1992). Although this is consistent with homicides in general, what is unique in these cases is that these involve predominantly male violence enacted upon a female partner and in many cases children, whereas most homicides in the United States involve male-on-male violence (Cooper and Smith 2011). Whereas only 18% of homicides in the United States involve the killing of an intimate partner, 72% of all murder-suicides involve an intimate partner (see Chapters 1 and 2).

In the Violence Policy Center (2015) study, 46% (or 6 of 13) of murder-suicides involved a male murderer and three or more victims. The study reported that many of these family annihilators had depression, often had financial problems, and felt the family was better off dying with them than remaining alive to deal with the problems (Abrahms 2005). Eighty-one percent of the murder-suicides occurred in the home. In terms of age of the murderer, one-third (33%) of murder-suicides involved a murderer age 55 years or older. This proportion of older perpetrators is in contrast to what is seen in other homicides, where the perpetrator is much younger, but is consistent with the larger percentage of completed suicides by men over 55.

The data collected in five different 6-month periods by the Violence Policy Center (2015) have been fairly consistent. Murder-suicides occur in the home in 75%–80% of cases and usually in the bedroom, and firearms are involved in 90%–95% of the cases. The killer is male 90%–95% of the time, and the murder-suicides involved intimate partners in 72%–74% of the cases. Interestingly, around 25%–33% of the cases involved elderly individuals, clearly a subset of murder-suicide as discussed in Chapter 9.

An additional way to explore the dynamics of familicides involves examining data on mass killings. Some experts consider familicide to be a subtype of mass killings. A recent study by Everytown for Gun Safety (2017) analyzed every mass shooting that occurred between January 2009 and December 2016 in the United States—a total of 156 mass shootings—by examining U.S. Federal Bureau of Investigation (FBI) data and media reports. These incidents, which the FBI defines as the killing of four or more people not including the shooter, resulted in 1,187 victims shot, with 848 killed and 339 injured. Sixty-six of the perpetrators killed themselves after the mass shooting; another 17 were shot and killed by law enforcement. One in four of the victims (211 total) were children.

This study showed that 50% of the victims were women and that the shooter killed a current or former spouse, intimate partner, or family member in 54% of the incidents (85 of 156). By contrast, women composed only 15% of total gun homicide victims in the United States in the studied time frame. This subcategory involving the killing of a domestic partner or family member accounted for 422 of the 848 victims killed in all mass shootings in the United States during this period. Forty percent of the fatalities in this subgroup were children. In a majority of these cases (56), the perpetrator ended up killing himself.

Forty-two percent of all mass shooting perpetrators exhibited warning signs before the shooting. Such behaviors as recent acts, attempted acts, or threats of violence toward oneself or others; violation of protective orders; or evidence of ongoing substance abuse were noted in these cases. This is in contrast to the narrower category of familicides in which it is common that investigations do not uncover warning signs that may have preceded the violence. Sixty-three percent of all mass shootings took place in private homes as opposed to public spaces.

MOTIVES AND UNIQUE CHARACTERISTICS

The category of familicide is a subgroup distinct from murder-suicides involving the killing of strangers or cases involving aging couples in which mercy killing may be involved (see Chapter 9). Attempts to uncover dynamics and thus provide meaningful information for risk assessment are hindered by the limited number of such tragedies.

Dietz (1986) described familicide perpetrators and coined the term *family annihilator.* He considered this a type of mass murderer along with "pseudo commandos" and "set-and-run killers." He noted that a family annihilator is "usually the senior man of the house, who is depressed, paranoid, intoxicated or combination of these. He kills each member of the family who is present, sometimes including pets. He may commit suicide after killing the others, or may force the police to kill him" (p. 482).

Wilson et al. (1995) contrasted familicide and family annihilation with the related categories of filicide (i.e., killing of children by parents) and uxoricide (i.e., killing of a wife by a husband). According to their work, one commonality in all three types of murder requires studying the dynamic of interpersonal conflict and asking the question "Why do some human conflicts lead to such horrific ends?" Studying the relationship between victims and killer can be useful in any attempt to classify homicides. In uxoricides, it is common that sexual jealousy in the context of threats of separation or abandonment are common dynamics. Because the vast majority of these murder-suicides involve males in intimate relationships, not surprisingly, most of these cases involve some type of breakdown in the relationship that leads to violence. These authors proposed that better understanding of the underlying marital conflict, parent-child conflict, and the overlap of the two may be one approach to understanding familicides. Their approach was to ask the question of whether the mind-set of the killer in familicide is similar to the mind-set of the killer in filicide or the killer in uxoricide.

Wilson et al. (1995) identified many cases in which the children are secondary targets and the spouse is the primary target of the killer's hostility. This would include the circumstance in which the child is defending one parent from the violence of the other parent and therefore becomes a victim. In another scenario, the child is assaulted or killed to spite or terrorize a spouse, who then is also attacked. Again, the violence to the child is secondary, and the spouse or intimate partner is the primary focus of the hostility. The authors concluded that familicide is more like uxoricide than like filicide.

In addition, these authors anticipated that familicides would involve killers who are more despondent or insane, because they hypothesized that in killing both spouse and children, they have acted counter to their biological and evolutionary interests, and thus preservation of their own lives becomes meaningless (Wilson et al. 1995). Using national archives of Canadian and British homicide cases representing more than 19,000 homicide victims, they identified 109 familicide incidents involving 279 victims. Looking at data from Canada, Wales, and England, men were the killers in 93%–96% of familicides in a 13- to 16-year span. In contrast, men perpetrated 76%–81% of spousal killings and only 48%–52% of nonfamilicide filicides in these countries during this period. Another interesting finding was that stepchildren were more highly represented in filicides than in familicides. Additionally, in the familicide cases, shootings constituted a larger proportion of deaths than in filicides, and the male perpetrator committed suicide in half of the familicide cases in this sample; again, a rate that is significantly above rates in nonfamilicidal filicides and uxoricides. (Dying by suicide by men who killed persons other than wives or children is much rarer.) Children tended to be older in familicide than in filicide cases.

In Wilson et al.'s (1995) formulation, the data suggested that familicide appears to have more in common with the murder-suicide phenomenon of uxoricide than with filicide. The authors proposed two rather different familicide scenarios, both involving themes where masculine identity and control are pertinent and "where a proprietary conception of wife and family" is relevant (pp. 286–287). In the first scenario, they characterized cases in which marital breakup and infidelity may be part of the dynamic. In these cases, hostility is apparent and motivates the murders. In the second scenario, they described cases similar to Dietz's (1986) characterization of a depressed and brooding individual who is facing financial stressors and possible humiliation and sees the only solution as killing his entire family and himself. In this scenario, hostility toward spouse and children may be absent, and the killer may see his actions as altruistic. Wilson et al. (1995) characterized these two scenarios as the "hostile accusatory familicidal killer" and the "despondent nonhostile killer" (p. 289).

Similar to this perspective, Hodson (2008) suggested two categories of family annihilators: "revenge killers" and "altruistic killers." His categories are quite similar to Resnick's (1969) early types of filicide, which conceptualized many filicides as an "extended suicide" in which the father has decided to take his own life and for various reasons and circumstances then takes the lives of the entire family. Hodson's description of the "altruistic" type usually involves a despondent father who believes that killing his children will spare them pain and that, when religious beliefs are involved, he is sending them to a better world. The "revenge killer," similar to Wilson et al.'s (1995) typology, is the "hostile accusatory familicidal killer" in their model. Hodson (2008) noted in his review of studies that very few of the fathers who kill their own children, and kill their partner or spouse, are psychotic.

Wilson, a criminologist, and two colleagues, Yardley and Lynes, reviewed newspaper articles from 1980 to 2012 that involved familicide in England (Yardley et al. 2014). Their research presented a different profile of such murderers. The authors included fathers who killed their child or children, some of whom did not kill their spouse or partner, and some of whom did not kill themselves. Their study cohort included all filicides, but not necessarily familicides or filicide-suicides. They identified 71 cases in which 59 of the killers were male, and 75% of these men were between the ages of 30 and 49. In their review, Yardley et al. discovered that the fathers who committed these acts were not men with criminal backgrounds. Many times, they were employed, and in many cases, the family was reported to have a community of friends and families around them. As with previous studies, the majority of the murders took place in the home. In contrast to data from U.S. studies, the predominant method of killing was stabbing, whereas in U.S. studies the predominant method of killing involved firearms. Because the authors used a broad definition of family annihilator to include all filicides committed by fathers, 81% of the 71 cases involved the father attempting or dying by suicide, a high-percentage outcome consistent with the concept of family annihilator used throughout this chapter. In addition, about half of their cohort killed their partner or ex-partner. In 96% of the cases, the father killed his biological children. In two cases, the father killed stepchildren, and in four cases, the father killed members of the extended family in addition to his immediate family members.

Yardley et al. (2014) also identified breakdown in the family relationships—including separation from children, financial stressors, honor killing, and mental illness—as primary contextual circumstances for these murders. Breakup of the marital relationship was noted as the primary motive in two-thirds (66%) of the cases reviewed. Mental health issues were noted in only a small number of their cases. An interesting finding in their research was that there were no instances in which the murderer forced the police to kill him, as suggested by Dietz (1986) in his earlier article. This is likely related to the fact that most police in England do not carry firearms. In addition, the portrayal of the family annihilator as an unhappy, frustrated man with a long history of failures was not supported by this particular review of cases. Yardley et al.'s review also dispelled the notion of the father who accidentally kills his child or children in the enforcement of discipline.

Yardley et al. (2014) offered a typology involving four types of family annihilators: 1) self-righteous, 2) disappointed, 3) anomic, and 4) paranoid. The *self-righteous killer*, similar to the "revenge annihilator," tends to blame his partner or former partner for the breakdown of the family, and thus, this is the justification for his motivation in seeking revenge. Central to the motives of this type of perpetrator is that the father feels impotent and not in control. Yardley et al. described this type as a man who has a very rigid, inflexible concept of family. Masculine identity is deeply tied to the male breadwinner concept, and the idea that he can be replaced and made inconsequential is unacceptable. The *disappointed annihilator*, similar to the self-righteous killer, has an idealized rigid and fixed conception of what family ought to be. Whereas the self-righteous man believes this ideal has been destroyed by the actions of his partner or spouse, the disappointed annihilator creates the breakup because he believes his family has let him down. He sees his family as an extension of his own needs, desires, and hopes, and therefore, when he is disappointed in members of the family, he initiates the ultimate destruction of the nuclear family. The *anomic annihilator* is a father who is highly attached to status and wealth, and when he meets with financial crisis, he lacks the ability to adapt and change. Humiliation, shame, and impotence drive the individual to destroy his family and himself. Last, the authors characterize the *paranoid annihilator* as someone who is responding to a real or imagined threat to the family and children, who believes he is actually protecting his family from an external threat by killing his family members, defeating the threat before that threat can destroy his family. All four subcategories are linked to masculinity and the need for such men to exert power and control at times when control and power feel lost.

Léveillée et al. (2010) studied 16 cases of familicide (here defined as the killing of the spouse and at least one child) between 1986 and 1998 in Quebec. They compared this group with 36 men who committed filicide. They found that in 68% of cases of familicide the perpetrator committed suicide. They also found that perpetrators of familicide were a distinct group, in which the men were older, likely going through separation, experiencing economic stressors, and more likely to use a gun in the killing of family members. Léveillée's group also found that 68% of those who killed their family had a history of depressive symptoms, and 38% showed borderline personality traits. The case of Steven Sueppel illustrates Léveillée's perspective: Mr. Sueppel was a 42-year-old bank vice president who was on bail while charged with embezzlement. After admitting his responsibility and leaving messages on voice mails for family members expressing his sense of humiliation and shame, he took the life of his wife and four children, and then after a failed attempt to kill himself with carbon monoxide poisoning, he drove his car into a concrete pillar and died when his van exploded in flames.

Neil Websdale, a professor of criminology at Northern Arizona University, has characterized these murders as involving rage, revenge, and sometimes altruism. He divides family annihilators into two groups: the "livid coercive" killer and the "civil reputable" killer (Websdale 2010). In Websdale's typology, the livid coercive killer is driven by rage. The person may be controlling and assert authority over the household. When the wife tries to leave with the children, in an attempt to reassert control and to counter feelings of humiliation, the husband perpetrates extreme violence. The civil reputable killer is close to the "altruistic" killer described by others. The father's identity is deeply tied to the family and his ability to provide. Suicide is his solution when the financial crisis occurs. He sees taking the lives of his children and wife as a perverse form of rescuing them from hardship and shame and from his suicide. Websdale found in his research that the livid coercive killer often has a previous record or encounter with law enforcement.

Hatters Friedman et al. (2005) studied records in Cleveland, Ohio, from 1958 to 2002 regarding the phenomenon of filicide-suicides. Their hypothesis was that in filicides in which a parent then takes his or own own life, it is more likely that the killing of the child was related to altruistic motives or that the parent was psychotic. Of the 30 cases, 10 involved mothers and 20 involved fathers. These 30 parents were responsible for the deaths of 51 children ranging in age from 3 months to 17 years. Although not all children in these families were killed, 80% of the parents killed or tried to kill all of their children up to age 18. Relevant to this discussion on family annihilation, 65% of the fathers attempted to kill their wives as well as their children, whereas no mothers attempted to kill their husbands. In looking at the totality of the 30 cases, 55% of the fathers but none of the mothers attempted annihilation of the entire family. As with other studies involving familicide in the United States, the predominant means of killing involved firearms. Previous child abuse did not appear in the records of the vast majority of cases. Eighty percent of the parents had a history of psychiatric contacts and/or symptoms of a mood or thought disorder. Twenty percent of the mothers and 20% of the fathers appeared to have delusional symptoms prior to the filicide, and 70% of the mothers and 50% of the fathers appeared to have depression or depressive symptoms.

In terms of motives, Hatters Friedman et al. (2005) concluded that 90% of the mothers and 60% of the fathers were motivated by the desire to alleviate real or imagined suffering in their children. Only 25% of these altruistically motivated killings involved psychosis, and in 75% of the cases in this subset, the killer was not psychotic. Acutely psychotic motives, without the altruistic beliefs, accounted for 7% of cases; however, in 23% of the cases, the authors could not detect a motive. In conclusion, this study supported the authors' original hypothesis that the majority of filicide-suicide cases involved altruistic motives, whereas a much smaller number involved a psychotic parent. Fatal maltreatment of the child, unwanted children, and the desire for revenge on a spouse were absent from this small sample of filicide-suicides.

Unlike previous studies of filicide alone, in which children younger than 1 year are at greatest risk, in the filicide-suicide group, the highest risk was to children in the elementary school age range. Hatters Friedman et al. (2005) found results that were similar to those of a Swedish study in which the average age of the children in filicide-suicides was 6.5 years, and 70% of perpetrators were fathers. Other studies support the findings from these authors that depression and suicidal ideation, ongoing marital conflict or separation, and sometimes illness in the child are noted characteristics in the perpetrator's situation. Financial stressors may also be active. Interestingly, previous domestic violence as a risk factor was not found in the Hatters Friedman et al. study. In addition, this study identified more of the altruistically motivated and fewer of the accusatory or despondent killers characterized in other studies, which is in contrast to what Wilson et al. (1995) found in their study.

LEGAL ISSUES AND CONSEQUENCES

In familicide cases, there is little legal aftermath, because the father has murdered the entire family, including his spouse and himself. In family annihilations, surviving relatives, friends, and authorities are left with the challenge of trying to understand these extremely upsetting events. Many will ask if they could have foreseen the violence. Investigators attempt to collect evidence and interview friends, coworkers, neighbors, and family. After first eliminating home invasion and possible robbery as explanations for the crime, they try to make sense of these events and look for warning signs or other information that may be useful in preventing another such tragedy in other families. In some states, there are domestic violence fatality review processes and boards that investigate and examine the evidence and details with the goal of further understanding the crime and preventing future crimes.

In cases in which the father survives, prosecutions occur. When psychosis or other mental illness is relevant in the behavior of the perpetrator, insanity and diminished capacity defenses are sometimes pursued. But as Phillip Resnick discusses in the chapter on filicide in this volume (see Chapter 6), fathers are seldom found legally insane. They are more likely to be convicted and receive longer sentences than women found guilty of filicide (Kauppi et al. 2010; Resnick 1969; West et al. 2009). In some cases, when a child survives, custody and access issues may be involved in the aftermath.

ASSESSMENT ISSUES AND PREVENTION

As with filicide, it appears that a considerable percentage of fathers who become family annihilators have evidence of psychiatric symptoms prior to the event. However, few have actually sought psychiatric treatment. Although some situations may be identified in a clinical setting, education about depression and mental illness, including its possible fatal consequences, which may include violence toward family members and a spouse, should be used to promote destigmatization and foster more open communication about these concerns before they evolve further. There have been tremendous strides in identifying depression in the postpartum period as a risk factor for infanticide. Improving understanding among health care professionals that parents who experience depression with suicidal thoughts, financial stressors, substance use, marital discord or separation, and the presence of a sick or disabled child as associated factors for familicide should be a component of prevention. Parents with suicidal thoughts and parents who appear to have delusional thoughts should be assessed for risk of harming their children. Health professionals involved in the care of adult men should be aware of the risk factors associated with familicide.

The phenomena of familicide and family annihilation involve a variety of contexts and circumstances; there is no "profile" that considers all possible scenarios. Certainly, increased awareness in the workplace of men with families who appear depressed or demonstrate changes in attitude and behaviors should be part of any explicit campaign to increase awareness of such tragedies.

Risk assessment tools have been developed to help assess for potential domestic violence. Women who have been threatened or previously assaulted with a weapon are at substantial increased risk to be murdered. Educating professionals that depressed and suicidal husbands—especially in circumstances of separation from spouse and children, financial stressors, and the use of substances—are a possible risk to spouses and children should be part of any prevention programs on this subject. Additionally, episodes of jealousy and expressions of anger and suspiciousness can be warning signs and should be addressed.

Meanwhile, the role of guns in familicides is well documented, and when data from the United States are compared with data from Canada, England, and Australia, it is clear that access to weapons increases the chance of bad outcomes. Restricting gun possession for individuals involved in previous domestic violence and gun possession for those with mental illness require further debate and discussion.

AFTERMATH

Familicide or family annihilation represents one of the most emotionally difficult types of violence for extended family members who are left to process the aftermath of these events. Relatives, friends, coworkers, and the community struggle with not only the losses but often their inability to understand the violence involved in such murders. How could a parent kill their children? How could someone who seemingly loved their family do such a horrific thing? Survivors struggle with the confusion and conflicting emotions, often needing to work through understandable anger toward the parent who caused the deaths while trying to accept the losses. With evidence that the perpetrator was depressed or perhaps motivated by financial or other stressors, survivors may be able to understand and even empathize somewhat. When information emerges that marital discord, perhaps separation and even infidelity, may be the underlying narrative, anger is inevitable.

In addition to family and close friends, the community at large often is confronted with distress regarding these cases because of the horror of these events. Such homicides trigger, especially when they occur in small communities, questions as to how more could have been done to support the family in trouble. Law enforcement examines previous contacts with the family, if any contacts occurred, looking for warning signs. The media may struggle with the sensational aspect of these crimes while recognizing that survivors should be respected in their desire for privacy during their mourning. The entire community is joined around, unfortunately, not a positive or hopeful occasion but a community tragedy; often, there are more questions than answers.

In some cases, the perpetrator may survive a suicide attempt that is unsuccessful, resulting in an extended legal process that brings the familicide back into public awareness. Communities may be divided in terms of attributing blame versus exercising understanding and forgiveness. Families are often divided. Relatives of the deceased spouse may solidify in their anger and wish for punishment for the perpetrator, whereas the surviving perpetrator's family may stand by their relative in the belief that mental illness motivated the tragedy.

CONCLUSION

After finding Brian Short, his wife, and three children in their home, police and the community struggled to find answers. Detective Mike O'Keefe, the lead investigator stated, "Unfortunately, we're never going to know the series of events that happened in that residence, we're never going to have a clear understanding of why" (Collin 2016). At the family funeral, Mr. Short's brother-in-law commented that Brian had been depressed and anxious, had lost considerable weight, and had tried several medications (Kieffer 2016). Ultimately, police investigators were not able to determine a clear motive.

Familicide and family annihilation are disturbing occurrences in our community. Research in the past 20–30 years has helped identify some common characteristics of the perpetrators and some common circumstances that may be associated with these horrible events. Clearly, the vast majority of familicides and family annihilations are perpetrated by men, usually a husband or male partner. Most of the familicides include the perpetrator's death by suicide or an attempted suicide by the perpetrator. The vast majority of these phenomena occur in the home and in private spaces. Depression, financial stressors, increased substance use, and threatened or actual separation from spouse and children are common circumstances in these murders. Various studies support the concept of two major categories of male familicide perpetrators. The first category, what some researchers have labeled the "altruistic killer," involves a depressed father undergoing financial strain who takes the lives of his family in reaction to what he perceives as "no way out" except in death. The second category involves a father who is facing separation and loss of family, whether imagined or real, who then reacts with anger and revenge. Attempts to create a typology of familicide or family annihilations have been challenging because of the variety in these phenomena, which may not only include killings of family members and the perpetrator but may also extend to the workplace, to school, and even to strangers and public spaces. Although there has been much variation in the research literature in identifying the motives of these murderers and providing a "profile" of such killers, it is clear that there is no profile that effectively describes this as a singular phenomenon. On the contrary, cases as varied as Charles Whitman's killing of 14 in the University of Texas tower shooting; Ronald Gene Simmons's killing of 16 family members and acquaintances in Arkansas in 1987 (he was ultimately executed in 1990 after refusing all appeals); and Brian Short's killing of his family and subsequent suicide, which is featured in this chapter, all fall within this category of homicide.

REFERENCES

Abrahms D: Finances, depression often issues for 'Family Annihilators.' The Desert Sun, May 12, 2005

Auchter B: Men who murder their families: what the research tells us. NIJ Journal 10:11–12, 2010.

Collin L: Lake Minnetonka murder-suicide still weighs heavy on small town police. WCCO CBS Minnesota, February 9, 2016. Available at: http://minnesota.cbslocal.com/2016/02/09/lake-minnetonka-murder-suicide-still-weighs-heavy-on-small-town-police. Accessed July 16, 2017.

Cooper A, Smith EL: Homicide Trends in the United States, 1980–2008. Trends by Sex, Bureau of Justice Statistics. Washington, DC, U.S. Department of Justice, November 2011

Dietz PE: Mass, serial and sensational homicides. Bull N Y Acad Med 62(5):477–491, 1986 3461857

Duwe G: The patterns and prevalence of mass murder in twentieth-century America. Justice Q 21(4):729–761, 2004

Duwe G: Mass Murder in the United States: A History. Jefferson, NC, McFarland and Co, 2007

Everytown for Gun Safety: Mass shootings in the United States: 2009–2016. Reports: Gun Violence Trends, April 11, 2017. Available at: https://everytownresearch.org/reports/mass-shootings-analysis/. Accessed July 16, 2017.

Felthous AR, Hempel A: Combined homicide-suicides: a review. J Forensic Sci 40(5):846–857, 1995 7595329

Hatters Friedman S, Resnick PJ: Parents who kill: why they do it. Psychiatr Times 26(5):10–12, 2009 Available at: www.psychiatrictimes.com/articles/parents-who-kill. Accessed July 16, 2017.

Hatters Friedman S, Hrouda DR, Holden CE, et al: Filicide-suicide: common factors in parents who kill their children and themselves. J Am Acad Psychiatry Law 33(4):496–504, 2005 16394226

Hodson P: Family annihilators: why fathers murder their own children. Originally published in Marie Claire magazine, September 2008. Available at: http://www.philliphodson.co.uk/family annihilators-why-men-murder-their-own-children-september-2008/. Accessed July 17, 2017.

Kauppi A, Kumpulainen K, Karkola K, et al: Maternal and paternal filicides: a retrospective review of filicides in Finland. J Am Acad Psychiatry Law 38(2):229–238, 2010 20542944

Kieffer P: Greenwood murder-suicide case concludes. Sun Sailor, January 27, 2016. Available at: http://sailor.mnsun.com/2016/01/27/greenwood-murder-suicide-case-concludes/. Accessed July 16, 2017.

Léveillée S, Marleau J, Lefebvre J: Familicide and filicide: there are two distinct realities? L'évolution psychiatrique 75(1):19–33, 2010

Marzuk PM, Tardiff K, Hirsch CS: The epidemiology of murder-suicide. JAMA 267(23):3179–3183, 1992 1593740

Morton RJ, Hilts MA (eds): Serial Murder: Multi-Disciplinary Perspectives for Investigators. Washington, DC, U.S. Federal Bureau of Investigation, 2005. Available at: http://bit.ly/1hWdFVU. Accessed July 16, 2017.

Newberger J: Behind the Tower: New Histories of the UT Tower Shooting. The Public History Seminar at UT Austin, 2016. Available at: http://behindthetower.org. Accessed July 16, 2017.

Resnick PJ: Child murder by parents: a psychiatric review of filicide. Am J Psychiatry 126(3):325–334, 1969 5801251

Violence Policy Center: American Roulette: Murder-Suicide in the United States, 5th Edition. Washington, DC, Violence Policy Center, 2015. Available at: http://www.vpc.org/publications/. Accessed July 16, 2017.

Websdale N: Familicidal Hearts: The Emotional Styles of 211 Killers. New York, Oxford University Press, 2010

West SG, Friedman SH, Resnick PJ: Fathers who kill their children: an analysis of the literature. J Forensic Sci 54(2):463–468, 2009 19187457

Wilson M, Daly M, Daniele A: Familicide: the killing of spouse and children. Aggress Behav 21(4):275–291, 1995

Yardley E, Wilson D, Lynes A: A taxonomy of male British family annihilators, 1980–2012. The Howard Journal of Crime and Justice 53(2):117–140, 2014

Conclusion

Susan Hatters Friedman, M.D.

From the cases of Susan Smith and the Menendez brothers to "black widow" killers and the "geriatric Romeo and Juliet," we have seen that familial homicides vary in nature as much as families themselves. Yet, a theme common to many of the cases explored in this book is that those who kill are often grappling with significant stressors, such as financial challenges, employment setbacks, and physical illness. Although mental illness plays a role in many deaths, it is far from the only factor.

The relationship between stressors and mental health is complex. Often the perpetrators perceive their challenges as insurmountable: the overwhelmed caregiver; the devoted father and loyal husband who loses his job and finds his role as "breadwinner" threatened; the depressed young mother without social support who turns to alcohol. Themes of anger, suspicion, or deep-seated resentment also abound in family murder cases. These may prove particularly noticeable in the intimate partner homicides originating from pathological jealousy; feticides in which the male partner kills to avoid paying child support or to terminate the relationship permanently; neonaticides in which the new mother wants the infant—"the problem"—to disappear to avoid a feared loss of family or status should her pregnancy become known; fatal maltreatment cases in which the child dies as a result of chronic neglect or abuse; revenge filicides in which one parent kills their partner's favorite child in an act aimed at emotionally wounding the partner; and siblicides committed out of jealousy or anger.

One must, in completing evaluations, consider the multiplicity of motives. Killings of a parent by mentally ill adult children stand in contrast to abused teenagers striking back; the latter may prove more similar to victims' responses in "battered woman" homicide cases. Older adult intimate homicides may occur either in the altruistic caregiving context or as an escalation after many years of ongoing intimate partner violence. Common emotions leading to motives for murder are seen in many pathological relationships.

Motives behind family murders, then, are often extreme versions of emotions that everyone has experienced at some point—anger, jealousy, greed, injured pride, or the desire for revenge. Occasionally, as in the case of the "black widow," narcissism or psychopathy—and lack of ever experiencing a loving relationship with the victim—appears evident. In other cases, such as in some feticides and neonaticides, a bond has not yet been established, and the perpetrator's concerns for his or her own self-interest weigh supreme. Much more often, however, significant emotional relationships do exist in which the family members have at some point loved as best they could—within the limitations of their own capabilities and life experiences.

In some cases of partner murder, child killing, and murder of a parent, the loving family member perpetrating the killing actually believes altruistically that he or she is doing what is best for his or her loved one. For example, this motivation may arise in the context of the victim who has a serious physical illness. Altruistic murders, as described in this volume, also may occur when the family member who kills is experiencing depression or psychosis. The depressed father and husband who holds a proprietary view toward his family may grow suicidal, but because he loves his children and wife and does not wish to desert them in a world perceived as hostile, he may kill them as well. The psychotic mother may believe that a fate worse than death will befall her child, such as that he will be kidnapped by a pedophile ring, and so kills him to spare him from that fate worse than death.

Prevention must be considered at both the individual and societal level. One-size-fits-all prevention efforts will not be effective because of the range of motives for the different types of family murder. However, knowledge about motives can help steer preventive efforts.

Men are more likely to kill their intimate partners than are women. A significant history of partner-directed violence usually precedes the homicide whether the death occurs in early adulthood or the golden years. Women who kill their partners fall into a range of categories, including not only abused women who strike back to kill their abusers and end the abuse but also the "black widows"; women with substance abuse or mental illness; women who possess the feelings of anger and jealousy more traditionally associated with male abusers; and, on occasion, overwhelmed caregivers. Women who kill their partner *often* act out of fear, whereas men who commit the same offense *often* act out of jealousy. However, as a society, we should be careful to recognize our gender biases and to question the assumption that men are violent and women are passive. As described in this volume, when women are violent, it is most often within the family.

Prevention of intimate partner homicide starts with prevention of intimate partner violence. It is the final fatal outcome, whether in the young or in old age. Prevention of intimate partner homicide by the abused woman striking back and of parricides in which the abused child strikes back similarly start with prevention of the abuse. The most frequent motive for filicide—fatal maltreatment—is the end result of abuse or neglect, and prevention of child maltreatment is invaluable in preventing the largest portion of child murders. Working backward, the dynamic (modifiable) risk factors for child abuse and intimate partner violence—for example, coping difficulties and substance abuse—thus need to be addressed.

Siblicide, rarer than other family murders, can begin, nonetheless, to be addressed by perpetuating the idea that although violence between siblings is the most common type of family violence, it is not okay.

Preventing murder of the newborn includes prevention of undesired pregnancy through sex education, availability of effective contraception, and safe abortions but also by making available options for safe relinquishment of unwanted infants—such as in Safe Havens, baby hatches, or anonymous birth options. In addition, considering what is known about young women at risk for denial or concealment of pregnancy, and later for neonaticide, building constructive relationships within the family and with trusted adults is crucial.

For altruistic filicides, prevention needs to target treatment of severely mentally ill patients who are parents. Family support is necessary when parents are unwell. Before this can happen, mental health professionals must routinely consider whether their patients are parents. Similarly, altruistic parricide prevention should include identification and treatment of mental illness as well as providing social support for mentally ill young adults living at home—and their supportive parents who face caregiver stress. Prevention of altruistic intimate homicide in the elderly may include careful screening for depression and burnout among elderly family caregivers.

It is our sincere hope that you have found the empirical data and clinical forensic experience discussed in this volume to be helpful. As this text reveals, family murder encompasses a wide variety of behaviors that stem from an equally broad swath of motives. There can be little doubt that mental illness, when present in these tragedies, is but one piece of the puzzle. Further research is needed to understand fully the context in which family murders occur. The limited research in this field ought not stop us from harnessing our existing knowledge in striving toward the paramount objective of prevention of family murders.

Index

Page numbers printed in **boldface** type refer to tables or figures.